THE LOW GI DIET REVOLUTION
and Other **NEW GLUCOSE REVOLUTION** Titles

■

The
Low GI Diet
Revolution

The Definitive Science-Based Weight Loss Plan

DR. JENNIE BRAND-MILLER
KAYE FOSTER-POWELL
with JOANNA MCMILLAN-PRICE

Recipes by Tracy Rutherford and Alison Roberts

MARLOWE & COMPANY
NEW YORK

Published by
Marlowe & Company
An Imprint of Avalon Publishing Group Incorporated
245 West 17th Street • 11th Floor
New York, NY 10011-5300

AVALON
publishing group incorporated

This edition was published in somewhat different form in Australia in 2004 under the
title *The Low GI Diet* by Hodder Headline Australia Pty Limited.
This edition is published by arrangement with
Hodder Headline Australia Pty Limited.

The GI logo ⒼⒸ is a trademark of the University of Sydney in Australia
and other countries. A food product carrying this logo is nutritious and has
been tested for its GI by an accredited laboratory.

Library of Congress Cataloging-in-Publication Data
Brand Miller, Janette, 1952-
    The low GI smart carb diet : the definitive science-based weight loss plan /
Jennie Brand-Miller and Kaye Foster-Powell with Joanna McMillan-Price ; recipes
by Tracy Rutherford and alison Roberts.
        p. cm. — (The new glucose revolution series)
    Includes index.
    ISBN 1-56924-413-8
    1. Reducing diets. 2. Glycemic index. I. Foster-Powell, Kaye.
II. McMillan-Price, Joanna. III. Title. IV. Series.

    RM222.2.B65 2004
    613.2'83—dc22

                                                                    2004058175

9   8   7   6   5   4   3

Designed by Pauline Neuwirth, Neuwirth & Associates, Inc.

Printed in the United States of America

Contents

Introduction

*I*t's time for a new approach to dieting. The Low GI Diet Revolution is a healthy, carbohydrate-controlled diet with low glycemic index (GI for short) values. It's based on choosing low-GI carbs, the ones that are slowly digested and absorbed, producing only gentle fluctuations in blood-glucose and insulin levels. Lowering insulin levels is not only a key ingredient in weight loss, but is also the secret to long-term health. Our own research, as well as that of others, actually proves that the Low GI Diet Revolution will:

- Reduce weight at a faster rate than a low-fat diet
- Decrease body fat, not muscle mass or water weight
- Increase satiety and minimize hunger pangs
- Maximize the metabolic rate during weight loss
- Reduce the chances of regaining weight
- Lower daylong blood-glucose and insulin levels

On this diet, you can eat sensible quantities of bread, pasta, breakfast cereal, rice, and noodles—it's just a matter of choosing the low-GI varieties. You will also eat plenty of lean meat, poultry, fish, shellfish, and low-fat dairy foods such as milk, cheese, and yogurt. Legumes play a starring role because they have the lowest GI values of all, so this is an easy diet for vegetarians to follow. You will consume generous amounts of fruit and vegetables, *except potatoes* (because they have a high GI value). Your salads will be dressed with vinaigrette made from healthy oils. You will eat three balanced meals a day, including a dessert or an indulgence at dinner, and we encourage you to have both a morning and an afternoon snack. You can even have an alcoholic drink with meals if you wish. And in the first three months, you will lose at least ½ pound of body fat per week: not water, not muscle, but pure *body fat*, most of it from around the waist. The scales can lie, but the tape measure can't.

This is not a low-carb diet, nor a low-fat diet, nor a high-protein diet: it's flexible and livable and, quite simply, it's a delicious way of eating that incorporates aspects of many ethnic cuisines. We promise that not only will you not be ravenously hungry between meals, but you won't be weighing out food, and you certainly won't be counting calories. One of the reasons this diet is so easy to follow is that it keeps you feeling fuller for longer. It helps control appetite by controlling blood glucose and stimulating the production of the body's own natural appetite suppressants. Metabolically, it reduces blood-glucose and insulin levels and maximizes the burning of fat. It is neither restrictive nor monotonous, and it includes your favorite foods. The Low GI Diet Revolution also has lots of value-added benefits: in addition to losing weight, you will reduce your risk of heart attack and diabetes, control your blood-glucose levels, and improve your overall health and vitality.

Written by internationally recognized scientists qualified in nutrition, dietetics, and fitness, the Low GI Diet Revolution is at the cutting edge of research on carbohydrates, the glycemic index, and weight loss. Our training and experience give us the tools to help both men and women beat the battle of the bulge. What's more, the Low GI Diet Revolution gets the nod of approval from nine out of ten nutrition experts around the world. Evidence that following a low-GI diet will help you lose weight healthily is published in the world's leading nutrition and medical journals. Even the GI skeptics admit that *The New Glucose Revolution*'s dietary advice offers a safe, balanced, and livable way of eating that puts no one at risk in either the short or long term.

The Low GI Diet Revolution is special for another important reason: it deals not just with energy intake (what goes in your mouth) but also with energy output—getting the legs, not the fingers, to do the walking. This is the critical side of the energy equation, the side that other diet plans largely ignore. Unless you consider this aspect, weight loss will *inevitably* rebound—if you weigh less, you need to eat less. It's that simple. But if you weigh less and exercise more, you not only reap the benefits of more muscle tone and *joie de vivre*, you can enjoy the same number of calories you did in the past without regaining weight.

We take you by the hand for those first twelve critical weeks of weight loss with a week-by-week plan (the Action Plan), advising you on exactly what you need to do and eat to get those pounds moving. Once you have completed the Action Plan, we don't abandon you. At this vulnerable stage, when you run the distinct risk of piling it all back on, we provide a three-point weight-maintenance program called Doing It for Life. Keeping the weight off is just as important as losing it, and it is essential to maintain the initial weight loss before you entertain any thoughts of losing more. Doing It for Life will teach you the skills you need to achieve serious, sustainable lifestyle change, the key to *lifelong* weight control. We show you how to embrace simple forms of physical activity and behavioral control that will keep your engine (your metabolism) revving and stop the yo-yo cycle of weight control. You will be taking care of yourself, looking good, feeling good, and maximizing your health in both the short and long term. Physical activity and healthy food habits will become just that: *habits* that are easy to sustain.

This is a family-friendly diet, too—your partner and your children, younger and older, will be sitting down to the same delicious food as you. Only the quantities will vary. Unlike other popular diets, this diet presents no long-term threats to bones, kidneys, blood vessels, or your heart; there is also no threat of ketosis or micronutrient deficiency. And if you are planning a pregnancy, this is the safest diet for you and your baby right from the time of conception. If you have found it difficult to become pregnant, this diet will increase your chances markedly, because it gets right to the root of the problem—insulin resistance—that affects about one in five women.

■

ALL THE ADVICE CONTAINED IN THIS BOOK COMES TO YOU FROM A TEAM OF EXPERTS TRAINED IN NUTRITION, DIETETICS, AND FITNESS, AND FROM THE WORLD'S FOREMOST RECOGNIZED EXPERTS ON THE GI OF FOODS.

■

WHO ARE WE?

Jennie Brand-Miller, PhD, is Professor of Human Nutrition at the University of Sydney. She holds a Personal Chair in the Human Nutrition Unit of the School of Molecular and Microbial Biosciences. Affectionately known in Australia as "the queen of the glycemic index," she is acknowledged worldwide for her expertise in the area of carbohydrates and health. Her series on the glycemic index, *The New Glucose Revolution*, has been translated into more than ten languages; more than two million copies are currently in print. Her research interests focus on many areas of nutrition, including the glycemic index of foods, diet and diabetes, insulin resistance, lactose intolerance, and infant nutrition.

Since 1981, Jennie and her team have played a key role on the world stage in establishing the scientific validity, benefits, and practicalities of the glycemic index. As such, she is eminently qualified to give you all the facts you need to put the Low GI Diet Revolution into practice.

Kaye Foster-Powell is an accredited practicing dietitian with a wide-ranging knowledge of the glycemic index. From measuring the glycemic index of foods at the University of Sydney to counseling hundreds of patients on its use to writing and speaking on its practical implications at an international level, Kaye is recognized in her profession as an expert on the subject. She has coauthored twelve books in the *New Glucose Revolution* series and compiled the world's first database of the glycemic index of foods, the International Tables of Glycemic Index, which have been instrumental to research on the relationship between GI values, glycemic load, and health. Kaye is uniquely skilled in her ability to translate her knowledge and understanding of the glycemic index into useful, practical advice for weight loss.

Joanna McMillan-Price, a nutrition scientist and a fitness leader, has the skills to help you change both your eating and exercise habits. Joanna has some thirteen years' experience in helping people get active and stay active, and she will guide you through an exercise and activity program that will help you to achieve a leaner, fitter body as well as better health, vitality, and long-term weight control. Joanna is well qualified to speak on the GI, having worked since 2000 with Jennie Brand-Miller at the University of Sydney on research toward her PhD, which compares the effects of diets varying in carbohydrate, protein, and GI values on weight loss—specifically body fat loss—plus the effects on other key health factors, such as blood cholesterol.

PART ONE

Understanding the Low GI Diet Revolution

Weight and Today's Diet Dilemma

*I*t's a sad but true fact that nineteen out of twenty people who lose weight by dieting will regain the lost weight. It's clear that a lifestyle solution to weight concerns, and not just another temporary fix, is needed. The Low GI Diet Revolution is about changing the way you eat for good.

Being slim, or of normal weight, is no longer the norm. Nearly two-thirds of adults in the United States are classed as overweight or obese. Men are worse off than women, and our children are affected, too—approximately one in four children weigh much more than they should for their age and height. Don't think this is just innocent "baby fat"—some overweight children are being diagnosed with a disease that used to be seen mainly in overweight adults: type 2 diabetes. Their lives may even be cut short or severely affected by blindness, kidney failure, or heart disease.

Even our pets are suffering—over a quarter of all cats and dogs are classed as overweight, and many have diabetes as a result. And our pets don't drink soft drinks, eat fast food, or watch television! Clearly, the origins of the obesity epidemic are complex.

Are you overweight, or just imagining it?

Women tend to see themselves as being larger than they actually are and to aspire to an unattainable size. Men, on the other hand, are better judges of their size, but often don't see excess weight as a health problem ("real men don't diet!"). To gauge whether you are overweight, get the tape measure out and measure your waist circumference—the smallest circumference around your abdomen. This point will be close to your navel but perhaps not exactly on it. Here's what you need to know:

	Overweight and at increased risk of disease	Very overweight and at substantially increased risk of disease
Men	Over 37 inches	Over 40 inches
Women	Over 31 inches	Over 35 inches

Astoundingly, the proportion of people with excess body fat has doubled in the last two decades—despite all our efforts to slim down. The food industry has met our demand for "diet" and "lite" foods, low-fat foods, sugar substitutes, fat substitutes—you name it, they've made it. But this hasn't stemmed the obesity epidemic. Indeed, some experts believe the food industry and its advertising are partly to blame for it.

Indigenous people such as the Aborigines in Australia, or those of Asian or African heritage, are at greater risk of disease even when they are only slightly overweight. For people belonging to these groups, at any given weight and height, there is proportionately more body fat in the abdominal region. This fat causes much more harm than fat stored in other places. If you belong to one of these ethnic groups, and if your waist circumference is over 37 inches (men) or over 31 inches (women), consider yourself overweight and at substantially higher risk of medical complications than people of other ethnicities.

We live in a push-button, "let-your-fingers-do-the-walking" era, and that means our food energy needs are very low—some would say pathologically low. Our current sedentary lifestyles require about 30 to 50 percent less daily food energy than those of our parents and grandparents. Fifty years ago, you were lucky if there was one car in the household—today there are likely to be two or more per family. Fifty years ago, television was in its infancy—now we watch an average of twenty-one hours per week. Surprisingly, eating only an extra 100 calories—the equivalent of an apple—over and above what we really need is all it took to tip the balance. That simple difference between energy in and energy out gave rise to today's epidemic of overweight. The good news, however, is that 100 calories can be burned up by just ten minutes of vigorous exercise or twenty minutes of brisk walking.

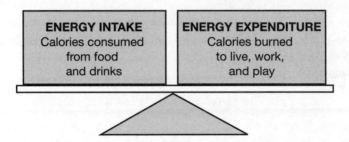

ENERGY INTAKE
Calories consumed
from food
and drinks

ENERGY EXPENDITURE
Calories burned
to live, work,
and play

Energy intake and energy expenditure need to be in balance to maintain a healthy weight. You will find it easier to achieve weight balance if the energy expenditure side of the equation is high, permitting greater food intake rather than the reverse. This is why diets that put all the emphasis on low food intake are doomed to fail.

Being overweight puts you at an infinitely greater risk of a range of health problems, especially type 2 diabetes. You also have double or triple the risk of contracting heart disease, high blood pressure, cancer, gout, gallstones, reproductive abnormalities, and arthritis. Being overweight even interferes with sleep, because fat around the neck area induces a dangerous form of snoring called "sleep apnea." So you become tired and cranky without knowing why. Along with this list of complications, there are emotional and psychological problems associated with being overweight. It can make you depressed, and depression can make you eat for comfort, ending in a vicious cycle. Medical intervention may be needed. Lastly, obese people are often discriminated against in employment situations, either consciously or unconsciously. And being unemployed only compounds the problem.

WHY TRADITIONAL, RESTRICTIVE DIETS FAIL

Chances are that you have already read several books and articles offering a solution to losing weight; miracle weight-loss solutions appear weekly. They are clearly good for selling magazines, but for the majority of people the diets don't work—if they did, there wouldn't be so many of them! At best, while you stick to it, a restrictive diet will reduce your calorie intake. At worst, a restrictive diet will change your body composition for the fatter. The diagram below shows the yo-yo pattern of weight gain and weight loss that is all too familiar to dieters. The overall effect of this pattern is a weight increase of from four to seven pounds per year. Why?

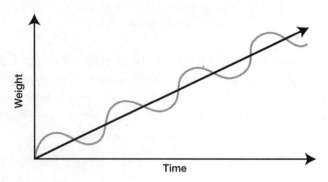

The yo-yo effect of restrictive dieting

When you lose weight through severely restricting your food intake, you lose some of your body's muscle mass. Over the years, this yo-yo dieting will change your body composition to less muscle and proportionately more fat, making weight control increasingly difficult. Your body's engine requires less and less energy to keep it ticking. This is nature's way of helping animals adapt to the environment in which they live—if food is scarce, then it is best to need less. The real goal in losing weight is to shed fat, not muscle mass or water weight.

One of the loudest messages in this book— despite its title—is: don't "diet"!

Don't severely restrict food intake, *don't* skip breakfast, *don't* skip meals, *don't* follow fad diets—you are just asking for trouble. Instead, we want you to adopt simple lifestyle "maneuvers," only some of which are specific to food. The aim is to maximize your muscle mass (increase your engine size), minimize your body fat (decrease the cushioning), and keep you burning the optimal fuel mix for lifelong weight control (high-octane energy with built-in engine "protectants").

HOW MUCH WEIGHT SHOULD YOU AIM TO LOSE?

Setting attainable goals is extremely important. You (and sometimes your doctor) may have completely unrealistic expectations of a weight-loss plan. You might be anticipating excessively rapid weight loss. A well-meaning doctor might encourage you to go back to your "ideal weight," a body mass index (BMI) between 19 and 25—the so-called "normal" range. If this is the case, both of you need to think again and to reconsider the rate of weight loss and the absolute amount you wish to lose.

To calculate your BMI, take your weight (in pounds) and divide by your height (in inches) squared, then multiply by 705.

Example:

A woman who is 5 feet (60 inches) tall and weighs 159 pounds would calculate her BMI like this:

159 divided by 3,600 (60 x 60) x 705 = a BMI of 31

A realistic weight-loss goal that still brings about desirable benefits in health and psychological terms is aiming to lose between 5 and 10 percent of your current weight over a period of twelve weeks. For example, if you currently weigh 220 pounds, then a weight loss of 11 to 22 pounds over twelve weeks is realistic and safe—and enough to improve your health. If you achieve that *and* are able to *maintain* that weight loss long term, you are a success! Furthermore, your risk of developing chronic disease is substantially reduced.

If you would like to lose still more weight, it is best to do so only after a period of weight maintenance. Your body needs time to adjust to a lower weight, so aim to maintain the weight you have lost over the next three to six months before attempting further weight loss. Each twelve-week period of weight loss using the Action Plan (see pages 57–67) should be followed by three to six months of weight maintenance as outlined in Doing It for Life (see pages 169–223), before you begin another weight-loss period. Using such an alternating strategy takes the pressure off and improves your chances of success.

What about weight loss in children?

One in four children today is overweight. If one of your children is overweight, don't think in terms of a strict individual diet program just for that child. Treatment of overweight children should involve the whole family. The Low GI Diet Revolution program is effective and safe for everyone. In children and adolescents, the emphasis should be less on controlling food intake and more on physical activity (the other side of the energy equation), particularly reducing sedentary activities such as watching television. We have given you some handy tips on page 214. Because children are growing, they seldom actually have to lose weight—maintaining their current weight (i.e., avoiding weight gain) should be the first goal.

What is a healthy weight for you?

Assuming that your weight is above that at which you feel healthy and comfortable, then it's reasonable to want to change. Let's begin by clarifying some details about why you might be overweight and what impact it's having on your life.

Place a check next to the statements that apply to you.

A. My weight (in pounds) divided by my height squared)   ❑
(in inches multiplied by 705 results in a number greater than 25.

B. I'm apple-shaped rather than pear-shaped   ❑
(i.e., I'm bigger around my waist than I am around my hips).

C. Both of my parents are overweight.   ❑
I have been big most of my life.   ❑

D. My activity level has declined in the past five years. ❑

I think I eat more than I need to. ❑

E. I suffer from one or more of the following:

elevated blood-glucose levels ❑

high blood pressure ❑

blocked arteries ❑

gout ❑

gallstones ❑

sleep apnea or snoring ❑

osteoarthritis ❑

shortness of breath on exertion ❑

My body weight stops me from doing things I would like to ❑
do, and which I would do if I were thinner.

A check at A suggests you are carrying more weight than is normally considered healthy.

Waiting to hear something you didn't know? What you have calculated here is your body mass index (BMI). It is a measure of your weight in relation to your height and is a crude indicator of body fatness in a population. It has significant limitations when applied to an individual, however, and should be used in conjunction with other measures of body fat in clinical assessment. In Caucasian people, a BMI greater than 25 is classified as overweight; above 30 is classified as obese. Clinically, this implies an excess accumulation of body fat to the extent that your health may be impaired. Different cutoffs apply for other ethnicities (see box on page 4), and more muscular individuals should use a cutoff BMI of 27. Bear in mind that the cutoff points are arbitrary, and that the health risk does not start at the cutoff point

A check at B implies an unhealthy distribution of body fat.

It is having a large mass of body fat that translates to health risks, rather than simply weighing a lot on the scales. So how do you know if you are actually "overfat?" Well, basically, you can see it, you can pinch it, and, if you are unsure, you can measure it. The simplest way to do so is with a tape measure. Wrap it around your waist, approximately at the level of your belly button. As mentioned on page 4, a waist measurement of greater than 31 inches for women and 37 inches for men indicates increased health risk due to intra-abdominal fat accumulation.

Checks at C suggest you may have a genetic predisposition to being overweight.

Scientists recognize such people as "easy gainers"—people who gain weight much more easily than others, thanks to their genetic makeup. Weight and body shape are largely the result of genetic background, as well as an individual's history of dieting and physical activity. Research suggests that those who have close relatives with a weight problem and/or more severe forms of obesity are more likely to have a genetic basis to their own weight problem.

Checks at D suggest lifestyle factors that might be contributing to your weight.

What lifestyle changes have you made that have caused a reduction in your daily activity? Did you change jobs, move closer to work, give up smoking (which slows down your metabolism), get a car, have an accident that immobilized you? Similarly, can you identify contributing factors to increasing energy intake, such as changed shopping habits, greater wealth, retirement, more reliance on take-out foods, etc.?

Checks at E suggest that your weight is affecting your health and your daily life.

It isn't true that to reach and maintain optimal health and personal happiness you have to be thin. Health and vitality come in all shapes and sizes. Rather, it is that deep, central body fat that we mentioned previously—what doctors know as "visceral" body fat (rather than fat just under the skin)—that seems to be linked with disease. Among these are heart disease, diabetes, high blood pressure, gout, gallstones, sleep apnea, and arthritis. However, excess fat anywhere on the body can still affect your health by limiting your mobility, causing you to puff and pant with exertion. The good news is that when an overweight person loses just 5 to 10 percent of his or her body weight and keeps it off, many of the adverse medical consequences of being overweight subside.

Unfortunately, most weight-loss programs, books, and magazines are based on the premise that people can control their weight and redesign their bodies regardless of physiology or genetics. The Low GI Diet Revolution is not about reaching a goal weight. It is impossible for you, or anyone else, to predict a healthy, achievable, maintainable weight for your body. Your chances of ill health are significantly lessened by losing just 5 to 10 percent of your body weight, as long as you stay active. A healthy, comfortable weight for you can only come about as a result of behavioral changes. By working through the 12-week Action Plan of the Low GI Diet Revolution, you will gradually develop the good eating habits and daily exercise pattern that will lead you toward a healthy weight for life.

YOU AND YOUR GENES

For a few blessed individuals, a constant weight is maintained year in, year out, without much conscious effort. Often, these people are naturally active and their body instinctively gravitates to a healthy weight. For others who are overweight, regardless of their efforts—every fad diet, every exercise program, even operations and medications—body weight is regained over the years. Why?

Let's take a look at the role genetics plays in weight control. There are many overweight people who tell us resignedly, "Well, my mother's the same," "I've always been overweight," or "It must be in my genes." In fact, these comments have some truth to them.

There is plenty of evidence to back up the idea that our body weight and shape are at least partially determined by our genes. A child born to overweight parents is much more likely to be overweight than one whose parents are not overweight. Most of this knowledge comes from studies of twins. Identical twins tend to be similar in body weight even if they are raised apart. Furthermore, twins adopted out as infants show the body-fat profile of their biological parents rather than that of their adoptive parents.

Are you an "easy gainer"?

If you have been significantly overweight for a long time, have relatives with a weight problem, and gain weight easily, scientists recognize you as an "easy gainer" and suggest genetics as the basis of your weight problem.

We also know that when naturally lean people are fed 10 percent more energy than they need, they increase their metabolic rate and their body *resists* the opportunity to gain weight—whereas overweight people, fed the same excess energy, pile on the pounds. The information stored in our genes governs our tendency to burn off or store excess calories.

Our genetic makeup underlies our metabolic rate—how many calories we burn per minute. Bodies, like cars, differ in this regard. An eight-cylinder car consumes more fuel than a small four-cylinder one. A bigger body requires more calories than a smaller one. When a car is stationary, the engine idles—using just enough fuel to keep the motor running. When we are asleep, the "revs" are even lower and we use a minimum number of calories. Our resting metabolic rate (RMR)—the calories we burn by lying completely at rest—is fueling our brain, heart, and other important organs. When we start exercising, or even just moving around, the number of calories (the amount of fuel we use) increases. But the greatest proportion of the calories used in a twenty-four-hour period are those used to maintain our RMR.

Since our RMR is where most of our calories are used, it is a significant determinant of our body weight. The lower your RMR, the greater your risk of gaining weight, and vice versa. Whether you have a high or low RMR is genetically determined. We all know someone who appears to eat like a horse but is positively thin. Almost in awe, we comment on their fast metabolism—and we may not be far off the mark.

Men have a higher RMR than women because their bodies contain more muscle mass and are more expensive to run; body fat, on the other hand, gets a free ride. These days, too many men and women have undersized muscles that hardly ever get a workout. Increasing muscle mass with weight-bearing (resistance) exercise will raise your RMR—and is one of the secrets to lifelong weight control.

Interestingly, we know that our genes dictate the fuel mix we burn while fasting (overnight). Some of us burn more carbohydrate and less fat, even though the total energy used is the same. Scientists believe that subtle abnormalities in the ability to burn fat (as opposed to carbs) lie behind most overweight and obesity. This doesn't mean that if your parents are overweight you should resign yourself to being overweight, too. But it may help you understand why you have to watch what you eat while others don't. One way the Low GI Diet Revolution helps is that it facilitates greater use of fat as a source of fuel.

Now, here's the kicker: the current epidemic of overweight can't be blamed on our genes. Our genes haven't mutated in the space of twenty years—but our environment *has*. So while genetics writes the code, environment presses the buttons. Our current sedentary lifestyles and food choices press all the wrong buttons!

Blaming Mom

Can your weight problem be traced back to conditions in the womb? Perhaps. Babies born with either a low (less than 5½ pounds) or high (more than 9 pounds) birth weight are at increased risk of health problems as adults. This is known as "fetal programming," and your metabolism might be insulin resistant right from the start.

So, if you were born with a tendency to be overweight, why does it matter what you eat? Well, genes can be switched on or off. By being choosy about carbohydrates and fats, you maximize insulin sensitivity, *up*-regulate the genes involved in burning fat, and *down*-regulate those involved in burning carbs. By moving your fuel "currency exchange" from a "carbohydrate economy" to a "fat economy," you increase the opportunity to deplete fat stores over carbohydrate stores. This is exactly what will happen when you begin to eat the foods we suggest in the 12-week Action Plan.

FOOD CHOICE AFFECTS YOUR APPETITE

Foods affect your appetite; they dictate when and how much you eat. If digestion takes time and involves the lower parts of your intestine, you stimulate natural appetite suppressants. Consequently, both quality and quantity of food are important for weight control. These are some of the mechanisms behind the success of a healthy low-GI diet for weight control.

Among all four major sources of calories in food (protein, fat, carbohydrate, and alcohol), fat has the highest energy content per unit of weight, twice that of carbohydrate and protein. A high-fat food is therefore said to be "energy dense," meaning there are a lot of calories in a standard weight of food. A typical croissant, made with wafer-thin layers of buttery pastry, contains about 480 calories—a whopping 20 percent of total energy needs for most people for twenty-four hours! To eat the same amount of energy in the form of apples, you have to eat about six large apples. So, getting more energy—calories—than your body needs is relatively easy when eating a high-fat food. That's why there has been so much emphasis on low-fat diets for weight control.

However, what really matters is not the fat content per se but a food's "energy density" (calories per gram). Traditional Mediterranean diets, for example, contain quite a lot of fat (mainly from olive oil), but are not so energy dense, because the oil is combined with a large volume of fruits and vegetables. On the other hand, many new low-fat foods on the market are energy dense. Indeed, some have much the same energy density as the original high-fat food, because 2 grams of carbohydrate have replaced every gram of fat. If a low-fat food has the same calories per serving as a high-fat food, then it's just as easy to overeat. Nutritionists have therefore had to fine-tune the message about diets for weight control:

- Eating more fruits and vegetables is more important than simply eating "low fat."
- The type of fat is more critical than the amount.
- The type of carbohydrate is important, too.

■

THINK ENERGY DENSITY PER SERVING— NOT HIGH FAT OR LOW FAT.

■

THE INSULIN CONNECTION

You are probably familiar with the hormone insulin. It is the one that is missing in people with type 1 diabetes and needs to be injected daily for survival. Most of us have the opposite problem—we have far too much of it circulating in our bodies at any one time. This is especially true of overweight people, those with type 2 diabetes or a family history of it, and indeed any man or woman with a "beer gut" or a "potbelly." Excess fat around the waist causes a form of inertia or resistance to insulin's action, resulting in the need to secrete more and more insulin to overcome the hurdle (a little like shouting to make a deaf person hear). These high circulating levels of insulin spell big trouble. The condition is known as "insulin resistance" (also known as the metabolic syndrome or Syndrome X). Probably one in two adults has this condition, but most of them are blissfully unaware of it. It is a silent epidemic, a ticking time bomb that sooner or later will erupt—most likely as a sudden heart attack, stroke, or diagnosis of diabetes. By losing weight, you can substantially reduce your insulin levels, especially if you choose low-GI carbs in place of your usual carbohydrate sources.

People with insulin resistance often have normal blood-glucose and cholesterol levels, giving them and their doctors a false impression of their heart health. But insulin resistance is at the root of most common forms of heart disease and diabetes.

We are often asked why insulin resistance is so common. The answer is that both genes *and* environment play a role. People of Asian and African origins and the descendants of the original inhabitants of Australia and North and South America appear to be more insulin resistant than those of Caucasian extraction, even when they are still young and lean. But regardless of our ethnic background, insulin resistance develops as we age. This has been attributed not to age per se, but to the fact that as we grow older, we gain excessive fat, become less physically active, and lose some of our muscle mass. Diet plays an important role, too. Specifically, diets with too much fat, especially saturated fat, and too little carbohydrate can make us more insulin resistant. If carbohydrate intake is high, high-GI foods can worsen preexisting insulin resistance.

The many guises of insulin resistance

If your doctor has told you that you have high blood pressure and "a touch of sugar" (prediabetes or impaired glucose tolerance), then you probably have the insulin resistance syndrome. If you're female and have irregular periods, unwanted facial hair, and/or acne, then you could have a condition directly related to insulin resistance called polycystic ovarian syndrome (PCOS). If you're overweight and *not* a big drinker but have abnormal liver tests (indicative of fatty liver), then it's likely you, too, are severely insulin resistant.

WHY INSULIN RESISTANCE
IS A BIG DEAL

Having persistently high insulin levels is likely to make you fatter and fatter, undermining all your efforts at weight control. It is the reason why people with diabetes find it so hard to lose weight.

The higher your insulin levels, the more carbohydrate you burn at the expense of fat. This is because insulin has two powerful actions: one is to "open the gates" so that glucose can flood into the cells and be used as the source of energy. The second is to *inhibit* the release of fat from fat stores. Furthermore, the burning of glucose inhibits the burning of fat, and vice versa.

These actions persist even in the face of insulin resistance, because the body overcomes the extra hurdle by simply pumping more insulin into the blood. Unfortunately, the level that finally drives glucose into the cells is two to ten times higher than what is needed to switch off the use of fat as a source of fuel. If insulin levels are high all day long, as they are in insulin-resistant and overweight people, then the cells are constantly forced to use glucose as their fuel source, drawing it from either the blood or stored glycogen. Blood glucose therefore swings from low to high and back again, wreaking havoc with our appetite and triggering the release of stress hormones. Our meager stores of carbohydrate in the liver and the muscles also undergo major fluctuations over the course of the day. When you don't get much of a chance to use fat as a source of fuel, it is not surprising that fat stores accumulate wherever they can:

- inside the muscle cells (a sign of insulin resistance)
- in the blood (this is called high triglycerides [TG], and is often seen in people with diabetes or the metabolic syndrome)
- in the liver (nonalcoholic fatty liver, or NAFL)
- around the waist (the proverbial potbelly)

High insulin levels are closely associated with risk factors for heart disease and type 2 diabetes. When insulin and TG levels are high, this automatically reduces the good form of cholesterol (HDL cholesterol), causing accelerated thickening and hardening of the arteries. High insulin levels also increase the factors responsible for blood clotting, thereby increasing the risk of blockage (thrombosis) in a narrow coronary artery and of a heart attack. Just as importantly, continuously high insulin levels lead to greater and greater degrees of insulin resistance, which leads to the need to secrete even more insulin. This escalating demand will eventually exhaust the insulin-making cells in predisposed individuals—just as shouting all the time eventually makes you hoarse. As insulin begins to fall, blood-glucose levels begin to rise, and the result is "a touch of sugar" (prediabetes), potentially followed by type 2 diabetes.

■

A HEALTHY LOW-GI DIET COMBINED WITH PHYSICAL ACTIVITY IS THE MOST POWERFUL WAY TO OPTIMIZE INSULIN SENSITIVITY AND DECREASE INSULIN LEVELS OVER THE COURSE OF THE DAY.

■

THE REAL DEAL ON CARBOHYDRATES

Carbs have gotten a lot of bad press lately, and you might well be confused about their value. You might even have been tempted to try a low-carb diet. Well, let's start with some facts about carbohydrate. Here are the advantages: carbohydrate is the most widely consumed substance in the world, after water. It's cheap, plentiful, and often sweet. Sweetness was important in our evolutionary past: it flagged a safe and palatable source of energy, so much so that "sweet" came to mean a lot of things—it was applied to love ("sweetheart") and to everything that made us happy ("sweet success"). Our first food, human milk, contains more carbohydrate than any other animal milk, reflecting the huge demands of the human brain. Glucose, the simplest product of carbohydrate digestion, is the obligatory fuel of the brain, of red blood cells, and of a growing fetus, and the main source of energy for the muscles during strenuous exercise.

Without carbs in our diet, we become heavily dependent on foods containing just fat and protein. That's not only unnecessarily restrictive, it's full of pitfalls.

Some human groups—the Inuit people of Alaska, for example—traditionally had few carbohydrates to choose from. Because of the climate they lived in, all their foods were animal foods, apart from summer fruits and berries that supplied small amounts of carbohydrate. They depended on marine and land animals to supply protein and fat for over 90 percent of their energy needs (there is little or no carbohydrate in animal food). We now know that there are limits on protein intake, because the human liver has a finite ability to metabolize the building blocks of proteins—amino acids. This ceiling on human protein intake meant that the Inuit and similar groups had a habit of craving fat, lots of it, particularly the blubber of animals such as seals and whales. But, and this is a big but, they were eating highly *unsaturated* fat, not the sort that promotes heart disease.

If we eat excess protein in the absence of fat and carbohydrate, ammonia builds up in the bloodstream, we feel nauseous, and we can eventually die. Indeed, that actually happened to explorers of America's West who, when times were tough, shot and ate skinny rabbits as their sole source of food for weeks on end. They eventually suffered from a condition known as "rabbit starvation" because, paradoxically, they were starving to death on rabbits.

For people in industrialized countries, avoiding carbs is a tricky business, because the alternative sources of energy are often high in saturated fat, and by eating them we run the risk of doing long-term damage to blood vessels and the heart. Indeed, there is more evidence against saturated fat than against any other single component of food. When people with diabetes were advised to eat low-carb diets in the first half of the last century, it helped control their high blood-glucose levels, but they often died prematurely from heart disease.

Nutritionists are also concerned that a low-carb diet will mean you miss out on all the valuable micronutrients that are to be found in whole grains, fruits, and vegetables. The vitamin and mineral supplements that are strongly advocated by the proponents of low-carb diets represent an admission that their diets are not balanced. What's more, supplements are not a satisfactory solution, because you still miss out on the protective substances that occur naturally in plant foods but not in pills.

LOW FAT OR LOW CARB?

There is much debate today about the optimal diet for weight loss. And not just among frustrated consumers, but among nutritionists and dietitians, too. On one side of the debate you have experts who consider a low-fat diet to be the best for weight loss. And it's true that liberal consumption of a low-fat diet leads to a small weight loss. But on the other side of the debate, Professor Walter Willett, head of the Harvard School of Public Health, and other notable experts believe that a low-fat diet based on any old carbohydrate is decidedly unhealthy. We agree. The reasoning behind this alternative thinking is as follows:

- Today's low-fat diet can be as energy dense as a high-fat diet.
- Carbs that are quickly digested and absorbed can stimulate appetite.
- Fast-release carbs will produce a marked increase in insulin levels.
- High insulin levels will compromise the body's ability to burn fat.

Proponents of low-carb diets claim that the best way to reduce insulin and body weight is to cut out the carbs altogether. They are right in some respects—you will lose weight much faster on a low-carb diet than on a conventional low-fat diet. But there is a catch: some of that weight is muscle mass and body water, not body fat. And while a low-carb diet might make you slimmer, you are not necessarily healthier. Indeed, you may be a step closer to a heart attack because you have substituted saturated and trans fats (partially hydrogenated vegetable oil found in some margarines, cookies, crackers, and snack food) for carbohydrate.

The burning question is *why* people lose weight faster on a low-carb diet. There are varying opinions among the experts. It could be the result of sheer boredom with such a small range of foods to choose from—you can't eat *any* cereal products, most fruits are off the menu, and sooner or later you can't bear the thought of yet another egg or piece of steak. It could also be related to the known appetite-suppressing effects of protein and high ketones in the blood (see page 35). It might also have something to do with the ability of protein to increase our metabolic rate, even though this effect is fairly minimal.

Our belief is that it has more to do with the drawbacks of a conventional low-fat diet than any special benefit of low-carb eating. Most foods that are 97 or 99 percent fat free are invariably high in carbohydrate, and increase blood-glucose and insulin levels. Furthermore, most people who are overweight are highly insulin resistant. Consequently, their insulin response to carbohydrates will be five or even ten times greater than that of a slim person. High insulin levels inhibit fat burning, and experts agree that bringing insulin down by any mechanism is one of the keys to weight loss. However, cutting out carbs is *not* the best solution. When you cut out carbs, there is a gaping hole to fill with just protein and fat. It makes food choices unnecessarily restrictive; furthermore, protein stimulates insulin secretion. Recommending a low-carb diet to reduce insulin reflects an ignorance of all the facts. It's overkill, and you don't need to go to such an extreme.

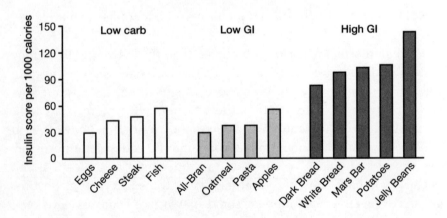

Low-GI foods have the same insulin scores as low-carb foods

If we look at the science objectively, it's clear that Dr. Atkins (the low-carb diet guru) was *half* right. High-carb diets that produce high insulin levels make it difficult to lose weight, forcing our bodies to burn glucose instead of fat. But as we have learned, carbs are not a homogeneous lot—there are high-GI carbs and low-GI carbs. Low-GI carbs produce much less insulin than high-GI carbs, because they are slowly digested and absorbed and improve the body's insulin sensitivity. Indeed, in our lab at the University of Sydney, we showed that acute insulin secretion after meals is no higher after low-GI carbs than after high-protein foods—the ones Atkins recommends in large quantities. For more information, see the previous graph.

THE BENEFITS OF THE LOW GI DIET REVOLUTION

You will be pleased to hear that there is a happy, healthy medium between a low-fat diet and a low-carb diet; that there is a diet that reduces insulin levels and increases the rate of weight loss without any potential to do harm in the long term. The Low GI Diet Revolution gives you the best of both worlds, the optimal balance between a conventional low-fat diet and a low-carb diet. Its emphasis on *slowly digested* carbs rather than *no* carbs means it is delicious, safe, and satiating, and reduces daylong insulin levels just as effectively as any low-carb diet.

The Glycemic Index: The Dietary Power Tool

*T*raditionally, the nature of carbohydrates was described by their chemical structure: simple or complex. Sugars were simple and starches were complex, only because sugars were small molecules and starches were big molecules. By virtue of their size, complex carbohydrates were assumed to be slowly digested and absorbed, causing only a small and gradual rise in blood-glucose levels. Simple sugars, on the other hand, were assumed to be the villains—digested and absorbed quickly, and producing a rapid rise in blood glucose. We now know that the whole chemical concept of "simple" versus "complex" carbohydrates tells us nothing about how they really behave in our bodies. Another system of describing the nature of carbohydrates and of classifying them according to their true effects on blood glucose was needed: enter the glycemic index. It took twenty-five years of scientific research—much of it controversial in the beginning—to prove that the glycemic index had enormous implications for everybody.

> **Low-GI foods have two important advantages for people trying to lose weight:**
> - They fill you up and keep you satisfied longer than their high-GI counterparts.
> - They reduce insulin levels and help you burn more body fat and less muscle, so your metabolic rate is higher.

It may seem surprising today, but scientists did not study the actual blood-glucose responses to common foods until the early 1980s. Since 1981, hundreds and hundreds of different foods have been tested as single foods and in mixed meals on both healthy people and those with diabetes. Professors David Jenkins and Tom Wolever at the University of Toronto were the first to use the term "glycemic index" to compare the blood-glucose-raising (*glycemic*) potential of different carbohydrates.

The glycemic index, or GI, is simply a numerical means of describing how much the carbohydrates in individual foods affect blood-glucose levels (*glycemia*). Foods with high GI values contain carbohydrates that cause a dramatic rise in blood-glucose levels, while foods with low GI values contain carbohydrates that have much less impact.

■

THE GI IS A MEASURE OF HOW QUICKLY CARBOHYDRATES HIT THE BLOODSTREAM.
IT COMPARES CARBOHYDRATES WEIGHT FOR WEIGHT, GRAM FOR GRAM.

■

This research has turned some widely held beliefs upside down. The first surprise was that the starch in such foods as white bread, potatoes, and many types of rice is digested and absorbed very quickly —not slowly, as had always been assumed.

Second, scientists found that sugar in foods (such as fruit, chocolate, and ice cream) did not produce more rapid or prolonged rises in blood glucose, as had always been thought. The truth was that most of the sugars in foods, regardless of the source, actually produced quite moderate blood-glucose responses—lower than most starches.

So we can discard the old distinctions that were made between starchy foods and sugary foods, or simple versus complex carbohydrates. They have no relevance at all when it comes to blood-glucose levels. Even an experienced scientist with a detailed knowledge of a food's preparation and chemical composition finds it difficult to predict its GI value.

■

FORGET ABOUT SIMPLE AND COMPLEX CARBOHYDRATES. THINK IN TERMS OF LOW AND HIGH GI.

■

THE KEY TO UNDERSTANDING THE GI IS THE RATE OF DIGESTION

Foods containing carbohydrates that break down quickly during digestion have the highest GI values. The blood-glucose response is fast and high. In other words, the glucose (or sugar) in the bloodstream increases rapidly. Conversely, foods that contain carbohydrates that break down slowly, releasing glucose gradually into the bloodstream, have low GI values. An analogy we like to use is the popular fable of the tortoise and the hare. The hare, just like high-GI foods, speeds away but loses the race to the tortoise with his slow and steady pace. Similarly, the slow and steady low-GI foods produce a smooth blood-glucose curve without wild fluctuations. To show you the difference we have drawn the following diagram, which shows the different effects of carbohydrates on blood-glucose levels.

For most people, the foods with low GI values have advantages over those with high GI values. However, for professional athletes, there are times when a high-GI carbohydrate will be the best choice.

The substance that produces one of the greatest effects on blood-glucose levels is pure glucose (sold as powder and in energy drinks).

GI testing has shown that most foods have less effect on blood-glucose levels than glucose itself. The GI value of pure glucose is set at 100, and every other food is ranked on a scale from 0 to 100 according

Carbohydrate
rapidly digested

Carbohydrate
slowly digested

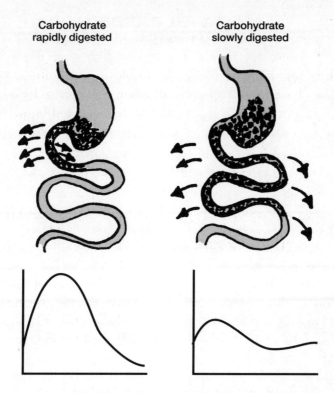

to the actual effect on blood-glucose levels. There are a few foods that have GI values of more than 100—for example, jasmine rice. While this seems extraordinary, there is a simple explanation. In testing, glucose is given as a highly concentrated solution that tends to be held up briefly in the stomach. On the other hand, jasmine rice contains starch that leaves the stomach without delay and is then digested at lightning speed.

Because low-GI foods are digested and absorbed slowly, they reach lower parts of the small intestine, stimulating the secretion of powerful "satiety factors" that help people feel satisfied. The Low GI Diet Revolution therefore harnesses nature's own appetite suppressants so that weight loss is easier to achieve than ever before.

∎

THE GLYCEMIC INDEX IS A CLINICALLY PROVEN TOOL FOR APPETITE CONTROL, DIABETES MANAGEMENT, AND CORONARY HEALTH.

∎

LOW-GI CARBS
HELP YOU LOSE WEIGHT

In our previous books we discussed the benefits of low-GI diets mainly in terms of appetite and blood-glucose control. Now we can argue confidently, on the basis of good scientific evidence, that the GI helps people lose weight—and specifically that dangerous fat around the belly we mentioned earlier. There is concrete evidence that a low-GI diet increases the rate of weight loss as compared to that of a conventional low-fat diet.

The confirmation comes from both our own weight-loss studies at the University of Sydney, as well as research from Harvard University and Hotel Dieu Hospital, Paris, France. We have summarized the evidence in the table on page 292.

What's more, some small but extremely well-designed studies have confirmed that the fat loss is maintained over the long term. That is a critically important point, because it is where other diets fail. Let's take a close look at all the facts supporting our healthy low-GI diet.

OVERCOMING HUNGER

One of the biggest challenges to losing weight is ignoring that gnawing feeling in your gut: hunger. It's impossible to deny extreme hunger—food-seeking behavior is wired into our brains to ensure that we survive when energy intake is too low. Extreme hunger followed by binge eating can develop into a vicious cycle—and that is one reason why we discourage rapid weight loss.

The Low GI Diet Revolution is based on an important scientifically proven fact—that foods with low GI values are more filling than their high-GI counterparts. They not only give you a greater feeling of fullness instantly, but they delay hunger pangs for longer and reduce food intake during the remainder of the day. In contrast, foods with a high GI value can actually stimulate appetite more quickly, increasing consumption at the next meal (as shown in the table on the following page).

When it comes to filling power, all foods were not created equal. Some foods and nutrients are simply more satiating than others, calorie for calorie. In general, protein packs the greatest punch, followed by carbohydrate and fat. Most of us can agree that a good steak has greater filling power than a croissant, despite the fact that they provide an equal number of calories.

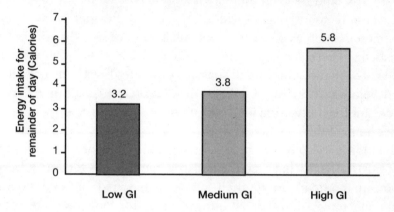

Low-GI Meals Are More Satiating

Voluntary food intake in 12 obese teenage boys
following test breakfast and lunch of varying GI

There are also foods that are "more-ish"—corn chips and potato chips, for example; we can't stop at one, just as the advertisement says. Fatty foods, in particular, have only a weak effect on satisfying appetite relative to the number of calories they provide. This has been demonstrated clearly in experiments where volunteers were asked to eat until their appetite was satisfied. They ate far more calories if the foods were high in fat than if they were starchy or sugary. Even when the fat and carbohydrate were disguised in yogurts and milk puddings, people consumed more energy from the high-fat option. This may surprise you, but remember: a gram of fat contains twice as many calories as a gram of protein, starch, or sugar.

In our laboratory at the University of Sydney, Dr. Susanna Holt developed the world's first satiety index of foods. Volunteers were given a range of individual foods that contained equal numbers of calories, and then their satiety responses and subsequent food intake were compared. She found that the most important determinant of satiety was the actual weight or volume of the food—the higher the weight per 1,000 calories, the greater the filling power. So foods that were high in water (and therefore the least energy dense), such as oatmeal, apples, and broccoli, were the most satiating. When water content was equal, however, protein and carbohydrate were the next-best predictors of satiating power.

Then, if carbohydrate content was similar, the GI became the most important determinant—low-GI foods being more satiating than high-GI foods. (It is true that potatoes, despite their high GI value, are high on the satiety index scale, but if we could invent a low-GI potato, it would be even more satiating!)

Invariably, foods that provided a lot of calories per gram (energy-dense foods such as croissants, chocolate, and peanuts) were the least satisfying. These foods are more likely to leave us wanting more and to lead to what scientists call "passive overeating" without realizing it. In developing the Low GI Diet Revolution, we made good use of these findings, encouraging food choices that will keep you feeling fuller longer.

In addition to our own research, at least twenty other studies from around the world have confirmed the remarkable fact that low-GI foods, in comparison to their nutrient-matched high-GI counterparts, are more filling, delay hunger pangs for longer, and/or reduce energy intake during the remainder of the day. There are several explanations for this, but above all is the fact that low-GI foods remain longer in the gut and reach much lower parts of the small intestine, triggering receptors that produce natural appetite suppressants. Many of these receptors are present only in the lower gut. It doesn't take a genius to appreciate that a food that empties rapidly from the stomach and gets digested and absorbed in minutes won't satisfy for hours on end.

In summary:

- High-GI foods may stimulate hunger, because the rapid rise and then fall in blood-glucose level appears to stimulate counter-regulatory responses to reverse the decline.
- Stress hormones such as adrenaline and cortisol are released when glucose levels rebound after a high-GI food has been consumed. Both hormones stimulate appetite.
- Low-GI foods may be more satiating simply because they are often less energy dense than their high-GI counterparts. The naturally high water and fiber content of many low-GI foods increases their bulk without increasing their energy content.

FAT LOSS IS FASTER
WITH LOW-GI FOODS

There are now at least ten studies showing that people who eat low-GI foods lose more body fat than those who eat high-GI foods (a summary of these studies can be found on page 292).

In one study conducted at Boston Children's Hospital, adolescents were instructed to follow either a conventional high-fiber, low-fat diet or a low-GI diet containing a little more protein and less carbohydrate. The low-GI group's diet emphasized foods such as oatmeal, eggs, low-fat dairy products, and pasta. In contrast, the low-fat diet emphasized whole-grain high-fiber cereal products, potatoes, and rice. Both diets contained the same number of calories and were followed for twelve months. At the end of the first six months, the people in the group eating low-GI foods had lost 6½ pounds of body fat, while the low-fat group had lost none. Furthermore, at the end of that year, the low-GI group had maintained their fat loss, while the other group had gained weight.

Diets based on low-GI foods prevent fat regain

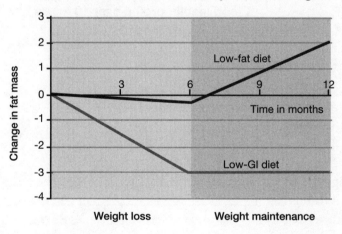

In our own research unit, we have made similar findings in a group of young overweight adults. To ensure dietary compliance, we gave them most of the food they needed for the whole twelve-week period. At the end, we found that weight and body-fat loss were 50 percent greater in those following the low-GI regime than in those following the conventional low-fat approach, as you can see on the opposite page.

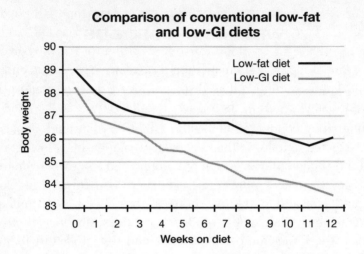

How did the Low GI Diet Revolution work? The most significant finding was the different effects of the two diets on the daylong insulin level. Low-GI foods resulted in lower levels of insulin over the course of the day, as shown in the figure below.

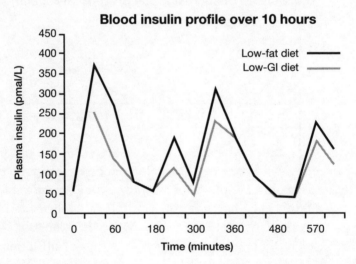

The hormone insulin is not only involved in regulating blood-glucose levels, but also plays a key role in fat storage. High levels of insulin mean the body is forced to burn carbohydrate rather than fat. Thus, over the course of the day, even if the total energy burned is the same, the proportions of fat and carbohydrate are different. Oxidizing carbohydrate won't help you lose weight, but burning fat will.

People who are obese appear to have high glycogen (carbohydrate) stores that undergo major fluctuations during the day. This suggests that glycogen is a more important source of fuel for them. If glycogen is being depleted and replenished on a regular basis (before and after each meal, for example), it is displacing fat from the engine. Each meal restores glycogen to its former high level (especially if the food has a high GI value), and the cycle repeats itself.

There are even more good reasons to choose the Low GI Diet Revolution for weight loss:

▶ When you first begin a diet, your metabolic rate drops in response to the reduction in food intake, which makes weight loss hard to sustain. Your metabolic rate drops much less, however, on the Low GI Diet Revolution than on a conventional low-fat diet. So your engine revs are higher.

▶ The Low GI Diet Revolution brings about a reduction in the dangerous fat—the fat around the abdomen—with minimal loss of muscle.

▶ Large-scale studies in people with diabetes have found that diets including low-GI carbs are linked not only to smaller waist circumference, but also to better diabetes control.

THE LOW GI DIET REVOLUTION
FOR LIFELONG HEALTH

One of the best reasons to adopt the Low GI Diet Revolution for weight loss and weight control is the value-added benefits you get for your long-term health. People who *naturally* eat a diet with a low GI or lower glycemic load (that is, the overall GI multiplied by the carbohydrate content) have been found to be at much lower risk of developing chronic and crippling diseases—the gamut of afflictions that adversely affect adults in the industrialized world. These include: type 2 diabetes, cardiovascular heart disease, and cancer of the large bowel, breast, upper gastrointestinal tract, pancreas, and uterus. The evidence for this comes from epidemiological studies based on large groups of people (10,000 to 100,000 or more), including the famous Nurses' Health Study being carried out by the Harvard School of Public Health.

What is the glycemic load?

The glycemic load (GL) provides a measure of the degree of glycemia and insulin demand produced by a normal serving of a particular food.

The glycemic load is calculated simply by multiplying the GI value of a food by the amount of carbohydrate per serving and dividing by 100.

GL = (GI value x carbohydrate per serving) ÷ 100

The glycemic load is greatest for high-GI foods that provide the most carbohydrate, particularly those we tend to eat in large quantities. Some nutritionists have argued that the glycemic load is an improvement on the GI because it provides an estimate of both quantity and quality of carbohydrate (the GI gives us just the quality). In large-scale studies at Harvard University, however, the risk of disease was predicted by the GI of the overall diet as well as by the glycemic load. The use of the glycemic load strengthened the relationship, suggesting that the more frequent the consumption of high-carbohydrate, high-GI foods, the more adverse the health outcome.

Don't make the mistake of using GL alone. If you do, you might find yourself eating a diet with very little carbohydrate but a lot of fat, especially saturated fat, and excessive amounts of protein. Use the GI to compare foods of similar nature (e.g., bread with bread). Ignore the GI of foods such as watermelon, cantaloupe, and pumpkin—they contain so little carbohydrate, it doesn't matter.

You will find both the GI and GL values of many foods in *The New Glucose Revolution Complete Guide to Glycemic Index Values*.

This type of study controls or adjusts for all the known compounding factors associated with disease risk: age, body weight, family history, physical activity, alcohol intake, fiber intake, and so forth. Hence it is highly unlikely that a low-GI diet is just a coincidental marker of a group of people at low risk for disease. The remarkable fact is that the GI and the GL often show strong relationships with disease risk while total carbohydrate, sugar, and total fat do not.

Furthermore, the GI values of self-selected diets have correlated in a reciprocal fashion with the strongest risk factor for coronary heart disease—your HDL cholesterol ("good" cholesterol). So if your diet has a low GI value, chances are you have a high good cholesterol value. That is an important finding, because nutritionists have struggled in the past to find appropriate nutritional advice for people whose HDL levels are low. Low HDL levels are also a feature of the metabolic or insulin resistance syndrome, which puts you not only at higher risk of heart attack and type 2 diabetes, but also polycystic ovarian syndrome (in women) and nonalcoholic fatty liver (more often seen in men).

Epidemiological studies also prove that many people are already eating a diet that has a low GI. In other words, it is practical and feasible to select low-GI foods from the vast array of foods currently on supermarket shelves. You don't have to jump through hoops or turn yourself inside out to adopt a diet that gives you the benefits of lifelong health and weight control. *The Low GI Diet Revolution* gives you all the information you need to make it happen for you and your family.

THE LOW GI DIET REVOLUTION IS THE LONG-TERM ANSWER

Any diet or exercise program can help you lose weight. But *maintaining* weight loss—not regaining the weight—is the real name of the game. Why go to all that effort if you put the weight back on again three months later? Weight *maintenance* differentiates the good diets from the bad ones.

Low-carb diets don't work in the longer term, because they represent such a huge departure from our normal eating habits. Most of us would find it simply too difficult to live in a modern world without our carbs and starchy staples, be they bread, pasta, noodles, or plain old rice. Avoiding sugars is twice as hard, because enjoying sweetness is programmed into our brains.

In contrast, the Low GI Diet Revolution is a diet you can live with. You will be as close as possible to your normal "comfort" zone while still keeping your weight under control. Fruit, yogurt, and even ice cream are part and parcel of our healthy low-GI eating plan, but are either off-limits or highly constrained on a low-carb diet. You will be eating the same delicious diet during weight loss (the 12-week Action Plan) and weight maintenance (Doing It for Life)—only the quantities differ. And it will be enjoyed, rather than suffered, by the whole family.

CARBS BOOST MOOD
AND BRAIN POWER

The benefits of carbs on mental performance are well documented. Glucose (from digested carbohydrate, or made in the liver) is the only source of fuel that our brains can use (except during starvation). The brain is the most energy-demanding organ in the body; it is responsible for over half of our obligatory energy requirements. Unlike muscle cells, which can burn either fat or carbohydrate, the brain does not have the capacity to burn fat. If you fast for twenty-four hours or decide to avoid carbohydrate, the brain initially relies on small stores of carbohydrate in the liver, but within hours these stores become depleted and the liver begins synthesizing glucose from non-carbohydrate sources—however, it has only a limited ability to do this. We now know that any shortfall in glucose availability has negative consequences for brain function.

Recent medical literature shows that intellectual performance improves following the consumption of a carbohydrate-rich food (or a glucose load). Tests carried out included various measures of "intelligence," including word recall, maze learning, arithmetic, short-term memory, rapid information processing, and reasoning. An improved mental ability following a carbohydrate meal was demonstrated in all types of people—young people, university students, people with diabetes, healthy elderly people, and those with Alzheimer's disease. Interestingly, it appears that low-GI carbohydrates enhance learning and memory more than high-GI carbohydrates, probably because there is no rebound fall in blood glucose. All of this evidence supports our belief that healthy, low-GI carbs should play an important role in your diet.

■

EATING TO LOSE WEIGHT WITH LOW-GI CARBS GIVES
YOU FREEDOM, FLEXIBILITY, AND SECURITY.

■

WHAT YOU SHOULD KNOW ABOUT LOW-CARB DIETS AND KETOSIS

At all times, our bodies need to maintain a minimum threshold level of glucose in the blood to serve the brain and the central nervous system. If, for some reason, glucose levels fall below this threshold (a very rare state called *hypoglycemia*), the consequences are severe, and include trembling, dizziness, nausea, incoherent rambling speech, and lack of coordination. When necessary, the brain will make use of *ketones*, a by-product of the breakdown of fat. In people losing weight on a low-carb diet, the level of ketones in the blood rises markedly, and this state, called *ketosis*, is taken as a sign of "success." The brain, however, is definitely not at its best using ketones, and one result is that mental judgment is impaired.

The Low-GI diet	Low-carb diet
You feel good, you can think straight	You may feel headachy and light-headed
You lose fat, not water and muscle Insulin sensitivity is enhanced	You lose fat, water, and muscle Glucose tolerance worsens
You have energy for exercise	You feel lethargic; exercise is tough
Low in saturated and trans fats	Unavoidably high in the bad fats
No concerns about safety in children	Immense concerns about long-term safety in children
No concerns about safety in pregnant women	Immense concerns about safety in pregnant women
Benefits for mental function	Decline in mental performance
Fits in easily with family and friends	Antisocial, often alienates friends/family
Value-added benefits for long-term health	Serious doubts about long-term safety

Ketosis is a serious concern for pregnant women. The fetus can be harmed and its brain development impaired by high levels of ketones crossing from the mother's blood via the placenta. Because being overweight is often a cause of infertility, women who are losing weight may get pregnant unexpectedly. Thus one of the very good reasons we advocate a healthy low-GI diet in this context is that there are absolutely no safety concerns for mother or baby. Indeed, there is some evidence that a low-GI diet will even help mothers control excessive weight gain during pregnancy.

We've summarized all the benefits of the Low GI Diet Revolution over a low-carb diet in the table on the previous page.

■

THE LOW GI DIET REVOLUTION IS NOT A FAD, BUT A BLUEPRINT FOR HEALTHY EATING FOR THE REST OF YOUR LIFE.

■

HOW MUCH CARB?

When pushed, humans can scrape by with no carbohydrate in the diet at all—your liver can synthesize most of the glucose your brain needs and use ketones to make up the shortfall. But you won't be operating at your peak either physically or mentally.

A low-carb diet is definitely not a good idea if you are trying to be more active—something we strongly encourage, because activity is *the key* to lifelong weight control. The more strenuously you exercise, the more carbs you need, and no serious athlete follows a low-carb diet long term (though they may use it for a few days to deplete all carbohydrate stores as part of a process called "glycogen loading").

What then is the optimal level of carbohydrate in the diet? Not so long ago, everyone was told that a high-carbohydrate diet (more than 50 percent of energy intake as carbs) was the *only* diet for optimum health and weight control. Thankfully, nutrition science has progressed since then, and we are now able to be much more flexible.

In 2002, the National Institutes of Health (NIH) advised that a *range* of carbohydrate intakes could adequately meet the body's needs while minimizing the risk of disease. Specifically, they advised the following ranges:

■

CARBOHYDRATES: 45 TO 65 PERCENT OF ENERGY
FAT: 25 TO 35 PERCENT OF ENERGY
PROTEIN: 15 TO 35 PERCENT OF ENERGY

■

We like these figures, because they allow for individual tailoring. The American Heart Association even ruled that you could eat as little as 40 percent of energy as carbs and not endanger your heart.

Chances are your diet already falls within these flexible ranges, and if so, we encourage you to stick with what you're doing. If your preference is for more protein and more fat than you are currently eating, then go ahead—just be choosy about quality. We believe that you are the best judge of what you can live with for the rest of your life, and anyway, there is plenty of room for flexibility.

If you have been making a concerted effort to follow a low-carb diet, your carbohydrate intake may be as low as 20 percent of energy. We believe such a figure is unnecessarily restrictive and possibly harmful in the long term, and encourage you to increase your carb intake. Because we want you to incorporate daily exercise as part of your weight-control strategy, you need your carbs!

We recommend that you consume at least 130 grams of carbohydrate per day, even during active weight loss. Nevertheless, regardless of the amount, the *type* of carbohydrate is extremely important. And that's where the GI comes into play.

THE SEVEN GUIDELINES OF THE
LOW GI DIET REVOLUTION

Choosing low-GI foods is one of *the* most important dietary choices you can make. As well as identifying your best low-GI carb choices, our seven dietary guidelines below give you a blueprint for eating for life.

> **1.** Eat seven or more servings of fruit and vegetables every day.
>
> **2.** Eat low-GI breads and cereals.
>
> **3.** Eat more legumes, including soybeans, chickpeas, and lentils.
>
> **4.** Eat nuts more regularly.
>
> **5.** Eat more fish and seafood.
>
> **6.** Eat lean red meats, poultry, and eggs.
>
> **7.** Eat low-fat dairy products.

■

LOW GI: 55 OR LESS
MODERATE GI: 56–69
HIGH GI: 70 OR MORE

■

1. Eat seven or more servings of fruit and vegetables every day

Why?

Being high in fiber and therefore filling, and low in fat (apart from olives and avocado, which contain some "good" fats), fruits and vegetables play a central role in the Low GI Diet Revolution. In addition to protecting you against diseases (ranging from high blood pressure to cancer), they are bursting with nutrients that will give you a glow of good health, such as:

- ▶ Beta-carotene—the plant precursor of vitamin A, used to maintain healthy skin and eyes. A diet rich in beta-carotene may even lessen skin damage caused by UV rays. Apricots, peaches, mangoes, carrots, broccoli, and sweet potato are particularly rich in beta-carotene.
- ▶ Vitamin C—nature's water-soluble antioxidant. Antioxidants are a little like your personal bodyguard, protecting your body cells from the damage that can be caused by pollutants in our

environment and that also occurs as a natural part of aging. Guava, peppers, orange, kiwi fruit, and cantaloupe are especially rich in vitamin C.

▶ Anthocyanins—the purple and red pigments in blueberries, peppers, beets, and eggplant that also function as antioxidants, minimizing the damage to cell membranes that occurs with aging.

How much?

Aim to eat at least two servings of fruit and five servings of vegetables every day, preferably of three or more different colors. A serving is about one medium-sized piece of fruit, half a cup of cooked veggies, or a cup of raw veggies.

Which vegetables are low-GI?

Most vegetables contain so little carbohydrate that they don't have a GI value. Potatoes are a notable exception, however—they have a high GI value. If you love potatoes, try to replace some of the potatoes in your diet with these low-GI alternatives:

Sweet Corn (GI 46–48)

Sweet corn contains folic acid, potassium, the antioxidant vitamins A and C, and dietary fiber. Add canned or frozen kernels to soups, stews, relishes, salsas, and salads, or simply enjoy it on the cob. For the best flavor, buy fresh corn with the husk intact, because the sugar in the kernels transforms into starch the moment the husk is removed.

Corn is often used as a base for gluten-free products. However, many products manufactured from corn, such as cornflakes, cornmeal, and corn pasta, do not have a low GI. Check the GI table first (see pages 269–88).

Sweet Potato (GI 46)

Sweet potatoes are an excellent source of beta-carotene, vitamin C, and dietary fiber. They make a great substitute for potatoes. Peel them or simply scrub the skins and steam, boil, bake, or microwave. Try mashing them with a little mustard-seed oil or wrapping them in foil and cooking on the barbecue. They also make a tasty addition to casseroles, stir-fry, soups, and (roasted first) salads.

Taro (GI 54)

Taro is a slowly digested food eaten widely throughout the Pacific Islands. It has a dry texture and a flavor similar to sweet potato, and can be used in the same ways. Before cooking, peel off the thick skin wearing rubber gloves (as the juice has been known to cause skin irritation), then cut into wedges and steam, boil, or bake.

Yam (GI 37)

Yam, with its thick brownish skin and creamy flesh, is high in fiber and nutrient dense. It's a good source of vitamin C and potassium. Similar to sweet potato and taro but with an earthier flavor, yam can be steamed, microwaved, boiled, or baked in wedges or roasted and added to salads.

Which fruits are low-GI?

Most fruits have a low GI value thanks to the presence of the low-GI sugar fructose, soluble and insoluble fibers, and acids (which may slow down stomach emptying).

The lowest-GI fruits—apples, pears, all citrus (oranges, grapefruit, mandarins) and stone fruits (peaches, nectarines, plums, apricots)—are those grown in temperate climates. Generally, the more acidic a fruit, the lower the GI value. Tropical fruits such as pineapple, cantaloupe, and watermelon tend to have intermediate GI values, but they are excellent sources of antioxidants and, in average servings, their glycemic load is low.

Most berries have so little carbohydrate that their GI value is impossible to test. Strawberries have been tested, however, and they have a low GI. Enjoy them by the bowlful.

2. Eat low-GI breads and cereals

Why?

What affects the overall GI value of your diet the most? The types of breads and cereals you eat. Mixed-grain breads, sourdough, traditional rolled oats, cracked wheat, pearl barley, pasta, noodles, and certain types of rice are just some examples of low-GI cereal foods. The slow rates of digestion and absorption of these foods will fill you up better, trickle fuel into your engine at a more useable rate, and keep you satisfied for longer.

How much?

Most people need at least four servings of grains each day (very active people need much more), where a serving is two slices of bread or a cup of rice or pasta.

BREAD

For most people, bread is an important part of the diet. One of the most important changes you can make to lower the GI of your diet is to choose a low-GI bread. Choose a really grainy bread, stone-ground or whole-grain bread, sourdough bread, or bread made from chickpea or other legume-based flours. Small specialty bakers are the most likely places to find such breads. Some healthy low-GI choices are listed below.

Whole-grain breads—Whole-grain breads contain lots of "grainy bits," tend to be chewy, and are nutritionally superior to other breads, containing high levels of fiber, vitamins, minerals, and phytoestrogens.

Choose breads made with whole cereal grains such as barley, rye, triticale (a wheat and rye hybrid), oats, soy, and cracked wheat, and that have seeds, such as sunflower seeds or linseeds, added.

Pumpernickel—Also known as rye kernel bread, pumpernickel contains 80 to 90 percent whole and cracked rye kernels. It is dense and compact and is usually sold thinly sliced. The main reason for its low GI value is the fact that it contains whole cereal grains.

Sourdough—Sourdough results from the deliberately slow fermentation of flour by yeasts, which produces a buildup of organic acids. These acids give sourdough its characteristic taste. This flavorful low-GI bread is a popular choice for sandwiches (its compact structure keeps the sandwich intact), makes great toast, and is generally considered acceptable by those family members who absolutely insist on white bread. The flavor blends well with all kinds of fillings and toppings, making it ideal for lunch boxes and snacks, and to serve with soups, salads, and main meals.

Stone-ground or whole-wheat breads—In such breads, the flour has been milled from the entire wheat berry (the germ, endosperm or starch compartment, and the bran) and the milling process uses a method of slowly grinding the grain with a burr stone instead of high-speed metal rollers to distribute the germ oil more evenly. Virtually none of the ingredients packaged in the wheat berry get lost in this processing method, and that is why this bread is such a rich source of several B vitamins, iron, zinc, and dietary fiber.

Fruit bread—The GI value of fruit bread is relatively low because of the partial substitution of wheat flour (high GI) with dried fruits (lower GI). The presence of sugar in the dough also limits the gelatinization of the starch.

Chapati-baisen—Chapati is unleavened or slightly leavened bread that looks rather like pita bread. It is widely eaten throughout the Indian subcontinent and is available in Indian restaurants worldwide. While it is often made with wheat flour, it can also be made from baisen or chickpea flour, giving it a significantly lower GI value (63) due to the nature of the starch. All legumes, including chickpeas, have a higher proportion of amylose starch than cereal grains have. So, before you order, ask what flour the chapati was made with.

Low-GI commercially made breads available in the United States

- Rudolph's Specialty Bakeries linseed and rye
- Shiloh Farms sprouted 7-grain
- French Meadow Bakery 100% rye and sunflower seed
- Alvarado Street Bakery 100% sprouted sourdough, barley, or raisin bread
- Arnold stone-ground 100% whole wheat
- Pepperidge Farm Sprouted Wheat
- Healthy Choice Hearty 7-grain
- Vermont Bread Company 100% whole wheat

BREAKFAST CEREALS

Traditional rolled oats cooked into oatmeal is about the closest most of us come to a true whole-grain cereal. Although many commercial cereals are labeled "whole-grain," the processing they have undergone has destroyed the original physical form of the grain. Some commercial breakfast cereals, however, still do have a low GI thanks to a less extreme degree of processing and the presence of other factors (such as protein or soluble fiber) that slow down digestion. See the list below for the best commercially available low-GI cereal choices.

Or try making your own muesli using rolled oats and a mixture of dried fruit, nuts, and seeds.

Commercially made low-GI breakfast cereals available in the United States

Kellogg's

All-Bran	GI 34
All-Bran Fruit 'n' Oats	39
Special K	56
Frosted Flakes	55
Toasted Muesli	43
Natural Muesli	40
Swiss Formula Muesli	56

OTHER LOW-GI CEREAL GRAINS

Barley (GI 25)

One of the oldest cultivated cereals, barley is very nutritious and high in soluble fiber, which helps reduce the post-meal rise in blood glucose and means its GI value is low. Look for products such as pearl barley to use in soups, stews, and pilafs, as well as barley flakes or rolled barley, which have a light, nutty flavor and can be cooked as a cereal or used in baked goods and stuffing.

Bulgur (GI 48)

Also known as cracked wheat, bulgur is made from wheat grains that have been hulled and steamed to crack the grain before grinding. The whole-wheat grain in bulgur remains virtually intact—it is simply cracked—and the wheat germ and bran are retained, which preserves nutrients and lowers the GI. Bulgur is used as the base of the Middle

Eastern salad tabbouleh, but can also be used in pilafs, veggie burgers, stuffing, stews, salads, and soups, or as a cereal.

Noodles

Many Asian noodles, such as Hokkien, udon, and rice vermicelli, have low to intermediate GI values because of their dense texture, whether they are made from wheat or rice flour. Lungkow bean thread noodles (GI 33), also called cellophane noodles or green bean vermicelli, are also a smart carb choice. These shiny, fine white noodles are usually sold in bundles wrapped in cellophane in the Asian food aisle of your supermarket or in an Asian food market. Soak them in hot water for ten minutes, then add to a stir-fry or salad, as they tend to absorb the flavors of other foods they are cooked with. They have a low GI value thanks to their legume origin (they are made from mung beans) and their noodle shape and dense texture.

Oats (rolled oats GI 59)

Rolled oats are whole-grain oats that have been hulled, steamed, and flattened; this popular cereal grain lowers the GI of oatmeal, muesli, cookies, bread, and meat loaf. Oat bran also has a low GI.

Pasta

Pastas of any shape or size have fairly low GI values and are great for quick meals. Served with tomato sauce and/or accompaniments such as olive oil, fish, and lean meat, plenty of vegetables, and small amounts of cheese, a pasta meal gives you a healthy balance of carbs, fats, and proteins. Cooked pasta should be slightly firm (al dente) and offer some resistance when you are chewing it. Not only does it taste better this way, but it has a lower GI value, as overcooking boosts the GI. While pasta is a good low-GI choice, a huge amount will have a marked effect on your blood-glucose level. Remember, a standard serving of cooked pasta is one cup, which may be less than what you are used to eating.

Most pasta is made from semolina (finely cracked wheat), which is milled from very hard wheat (durum) with a high protein content. There is some evidence that thicker types of pasta have a lower GI value than thinner types because of the denser consistency and perhaps because they cook more slowly and are less likely to be overcooked. Adding egg to fresh pasta lowers the GI by increasing the protein content.

Note: Canned spaghetti has a higher GI value than other types of pasta.

Rice

Rice can have a high GI value (80–109) or a low GI value (50–55) depending on the variety and, in particular, on its amylose content.

Basmati rice (GI 58), Uncle Ben's converted, long-grain rice (GI 50), and Uncle Ben's long-grain and wild rice blend (GI 54) contain higher proportions of amylose (a type of starch that we digest more slowly) than other kinds of rice, which produces a lower glycemic response. It is also more compact in structure and more slowly digested. *Koshihikari* rice, eaten all over Japan, is a short-grain variety with a low GI value (48).

Waxy or glutinous rice, often used for rice desserts as it becomes sticky when cooked, has a high GI. Arborio rice, which is especially good for making Italian risotto, releases its starch during cooking and has a high GI value as a result. Eat less of these kinds of rice.

> **Sushi (GI 48)**—These bite-size parcels of raw or smoked fish, chicken, tofu, and/or pickled, raw, or cooked vegetables, wrapped in seaweed with rice that has been seasoned with vinegar, salt, and sugar, make ideal snacks and light meals. Even though the rice used to make sushi can sometimes be short-grain and somewhat sticky, sushi still has a low GI value (in Japan they use *koshihikari*, GI 48). In addition, sushi made with salmon and tuna boosts your intake of the healthy omega-3 fats.

Rye (GI 34)

Whole-kernel rye is used to make certain breads, including pumpernickel and some crispbreads. Rye flakes can be used as you would use rolled oats: you can eat them as a cooked cereal or sprinkle them over bread before you bake it.

Whole-wheat kernels (GI 41)

Wheat provides a staple food to half the world's population. Soak whole wheat overnight and then simmer for about an hour to use as a base for pilaf. Some people enjoy wheat bran as a cooked breakfast cereal. Cream of wheat is made from very fine semolina; you can use it as a breakfast cereal or in puddings, custards, soufflés, and soups.

3. Eat more legumes, including soybeans, chickpeas, and lentils

Why?

Look no further than legumes for a low-GI food that is easy on the wallet, versatile, filling, nutritious, and low in calories. Legumes are high in fiber, too—both soluble and insoluble—and are packed with nutrients, providing a valuable source of protein, carbohydrate, B vitamins, folic acid, iron, zinc, and magnesium. Whether you buy dried beans, lentils, and chickpeas and cook them yourself at home, or opt for the very convenient, time-saving canned varieties, you are choosing one of nature's lowest-GI foods.

Legumes have two particularly useful properties among their armory of health benefits. The first is their content of phytochemicals—natural plant chemicals that possess antiviral, antifungal, antibacterial, and anti-cancer properties. Plus, legumes are prebiotics. This means that they provide food for our gut bacteria or "intestinal flora," keeping our digestive system healthy.

A bean meal doesn't always have to be strictly vegetarian—try using beans in place of grains or potatoes. You could try serving a bean salsa with fish or cannellini-bean purée with grilled meat. Butter beans can also make a delicious potato substitute. Although they will keep indefinitely, it is best to use dried legumes within one year of purchase.

How much?

At least twice a week as a main meal—such as bean soup, chickpea curry, or lentil patties—or as a light meal, such a mixed-bean salad or pea and ham soup.

BEANS

When you add beans to meals and snacks, you reduce the overall GI of your diet and gain important health benefits. Beans are available dried or in cans. Young beans cook faster than old ones and will also be more vividly colored. Substitute one 14-ounce can of beans for three-quarters of a cup of dried beans. Dried beans usually have a lower GI value than canned beans, but using cans is infinitely more convenient and the GI is still low.

Baked beans—GI 49

Black-eyed beans—GI 42

Butter beans—GI 31

Cannellini beans—GI 31

Haricot beans—GI 33

Lima beans—GI 32

Mung beans—GI 39

Red kidney beans—GI 36

Dried legume preparation

1 **Soak.** Place legumes in a saucepan and cover them with two to three times their volume of cold water. Soak them overnight or during the day.

Shortcut: Rather than soaking overnight, add three times the volume of water to rinsed beans, bring to a boil for a few minutes, then remove from heat and let soak for an hour. Drain, add fresh water, then cook as usual.

2 **Cook.** Drain off the soaking water, adding two to three times the volume of water as beans. Bring the water to a boil, then simmer until beans are tender. Use the directions on the packet or the information below as a time guide.

Don't add salt to the cooking water—it slows down water absorption so cooking takes longer.

Don't cook beans in the water they have soaked in. Substances that contribute to flatulence are leached from the beans into the soaking and cooking waters.

Shortcuts: Precooked canned legumes make cooking with beans quick and easy. Legume-based meals come together much faster than those based on meat.

Precook your own dried legumes and freeze them in small batches. You can keep soaked or cooked beans in an airtight container for several days in the fridge.

CHICKPEAS (GI 28)

These large, caramel-colored legumes are popular in Middle Eastern and Mediterranean dishes. You can buy them in cans or as dried beans. To cook chickpeas, first place them in a bowl, cover them with plenty of cold water, and soak them overnight. Next day, drain the water, then put the chickpeas in a saucepan and cover them with clean water. Bring the beans to a boil for ten minutes, then simmer for 1½ hours until they're tender.

You can also roast and salt whole chickpeas for a delicious snack food. Ground chickpea flour, also called *baisen,* is used to make unleavened Indian bread.

LENTILS (GI 26)

Lentils are rich in protein, fiber, and B vitamins. All colors and types have a similarly low GI value, which is increased slightly if you opt to buy them canned and add them at the end of cooking. Lentils are one food that people with diabetes should learn to love—they can eat them until the cows come home. In fact, we have found that no matter how much of them people eat, they have only a small effect on blood-glucose levels. Lentils have a fairly bland, earthy flavor and are best prepared with onions, garlic, and spices. Use them as a "bed" for grilled fish or meat. They are great for thickening any kind of soup or extending meat casseroles.

Channa dal (also called Bengal gram dal) are husked, split, and polished Bengal gram (GI 11), the most common type of gram lentil in India. They are often cooked with a pinch of asafetida (an Indian spice) to make them easier to digest.

SOYBEANS (GI 14)

Soybeans and soy products have been a staple part of Asian diets for thousands of years and are an excellent source of protein. They are also rich in fiber, iron, zinc, and vitamin B. They are lower in carbohydrate and higher in fat than other legumes, but the majority of the fat is polyunsaturated. Soy is also a rich source of phytochemicals, and in particular of phytoestrogens, which are plant estrogens with a structure similar to the female hormone estrogen. Some studies link phytoestrogens with improvements in blood-cholesterol levels, relief from menopausal symptoms, and lower rates of cancer.

SPLIT PEAS (GI 32)

Split peas are prepared from a variety of the common garden pea with the husk removed. They may be yellow or green. They take about an hour to cook after soaking and are traditionally used in pea and ham soups or for making an Indian dal.

4. Eat nuts more regularly

Why?

Although nuts are high in fat, it is mainly polyunsaturated and monounsaturated fat, so they make a healthy substitute for less nutritious highly saturated fat snacks, such as potato chips, chocolate, and cookies.

Nuts are one of the richest sources of vitamin E, which, with the selenium they contain, works as an antioxidant. Selenium helps guard against harmful UV rays to reduce damage caused by the sun and premature aging of your skin.

How much?

Aim for a small handful of nuts (1 ounce) most days.

Here are some easy ways to eat more nuts:

▶ Use nuts and seeds in food preparation. For example, use toasted cashews or sesame seeds in a chicken stir-fry; sprinkle walnuts or pine nuts over a salad; top fruity desserts or granola with almonds.

▶ Use hazelnut spread on bread, or try peanut, almond, or cashew butter rather than butter or margarine.

▶ Sprinkle a mixture of ground nuts and linseeds over cereals or salads, or add to baked goods such as muffins.

5. Eat more fish and seafood

Why?

Fish does not have a GI value, as it is a source of protein, not carbohydrate. Increased fish consumption is linked to a reduced risk of coronary heart disease, improvements in mood, lower rates of depression, better blood-fat levels, and enhanced immunity. Just one serving of fish per week may reduce the risk of a fatal heart attack by 40 percent. The likely protective components of fish are the very long-chain omega-3 fatty acids. Our bodies make only small amounts of these fatty acids, and so we rely on dietary sources, especially seafood, for them.

How much?

One to three meals of fish each week.

Which fish is best?

- Oily fish, which tend to have dark-colored flesh and a strong flavor, are the richest source of omega-3 fats.
- Canned salmon, sardines, mackerel, and, to a lesser extent, tuna, are all very rich sources of omega-3s; look for canned fish packed in water, canola oil, olive oil, tomato sauce, or brine, and drain well.
- Fresh fish with higher levels of omega-3s are: Atlantic salmon and smoked salmon; Atlantic and Pacific mackerel; bluefin tuna; and swordfish. Eastern and Pacific oysters and squid (calamari) are also rich sources.

Mercury in fish

Due to the risk of high levels of mercury in certain species of fish, the Food and Drug Administration (FDA) recently advised that although pregnant women, nursing mothers, women planning a pregnancy, and young children can consume a variety of fish as part of a healthy diet, they should avoid the consumption of certain species. Shark, swordfish, king mackerel, and tilefish should not be consumed, because these long-lived larger fish contain the highest levels of mercury. Pregnant women should select a variety of other kinds of fish—shellfish, canned fish such as light tuna, smaller ocean fish, or farm-raised fish. The FDA says you can safely eat up to 12 ounces of cooked fish per week, with a typical serving size being 3 to 6 ounces.

6. Eat lean red meats, poultry, and eggs

Why?

Again, these foods do not have a GI value, because they are protein, not carbohydrate. Red meat is the best source of iron (the nutrient used for carrying oxygen in our blood) you can get.

Good iron status can increase energy levels and improve our exercise tolerance. While adequate iron can be obtained from a vegetarian diet, women particularly must select foods carefully to prevent iron deficiency. A chronic shortage of iron leads to anemia, with symptoms including pale skin, excessive tiredness, breathlessness, irritability, and decreased attention span.

How much?

We suggest eating lean meat two or three times a week and accompanying it with a salad or vegetables. A portion of 3½ ounces of lean meat as part of a balanced diet will meet the daily nutrient needs of an adult, but larger amounts can also be part of a healthy diet. A couple of eggs or 4 ounces of skinless chicken provide options for variety once or twice a week.

7. Eat low-fat dairy products

Why?

Milk, cheese, ice cream, yogurt, buttermilk, and custard are the richest sources of calcium in our diet. Calcium is vital in many bodily functions, so if we don't get enough in our diet, the body will draw it out of our bones. This bone loss over a number of years may lead to osteoporosis and loss of height, curvature of the spine, and peridontal disease (deterioration of bones supporting the teeth). By replacing full-fat dairy foods with reduced-fat, low-fat, or fat-free versions, you will reduce your saturated-fat intake and actually boost your calcium intake. Plus, new research shows that calcium and other components in dairy products play a vital role in burning fat.

How much?

To meet calcium requirements, experts recommend that adults eat two to three servings of dairy products every day. Good low-fat dairy choices include skim, fat-free, or low-fat milk and fat-free or low-fat yogurts. A serving is a cup of milk, 1 ounce of cheese, or 8 ounces of yogurt.

If you're lactose intolerant, you can still eat yogurt and cheese. You can also try lactose-reduced milk, high-calcium soy milk, salmon (canned, with bones), high-calcium tofu, calcium-fortified breakfast cereal, and dried figs—all great-tasting non-dairy sources of calcium.

MILK (GI 27)

Milk is a rich source of protein and vitamin B_2 (riboflavin). As whole milk is also a rich source of saturated fat, choose low-fat and fat-free milk and milk products. The surprisingly low GI of milk is a result of the combination of the moderate GI of the lactose (milk sugar) plus the effect of the milk protein, which forms a soft curd in the stomach and slows down the rate of stomach emptying.

YOGURT (GI 19–50)

Yogurt is rich in calcium, riboflavin, and protein. Low-fat natural yogurt provides the most calcium for the fewest calories. The combination of yogurt's acidity and high protein content contributes to its low GI value. Fruit yogurts made with a sugar-sweetened fruit syrup have a GI of around 33, whereas artificially sweetened yogurts have a GI of around 14.

LOW-FAT ICE CREAM (GI 37–49)

Low-fat ice cream is a delicious source of all the goodies found in milk. It is important that you choose a low-fat (less than 3 grams of fat per 100 grams) variety for regular consumption so that you don't overdo your saturated-fat intake. Save the gourmet varieties for an occasional indulgence. Ice cream has a slightly higher GI than milk because of the presence of sucrose and glucose in addition to lactose.

The Other Side of the Energy Equation

*L*et's be blunt. If you don't build physical activity into your days, you have very little chance of changing your body shape for life. You can certainly lose weight through dieting alone, but chances are you will regain any weight lost (and probably gain more) over the weeks and months after you stop actively "dieting."

■

THE PEOPLE MOST LIKELY TO KEEP THE WEIGHT OFF ARE THOSE WHO RAISE THEIR ACTIVITY LEVELS AND MAKE EXERCISE A NATURAL PART OF THEIR LIFE.

■

HOW CAN EXERCISE HELP BREAK THE DIETING CYCLE?

Exercising while you lose weight will help you to maximize fat loss and minimize lean-muscle loss. This means you get *leaner faster*. Since you maintain or even build muscle, you can help to prevent the drop in your metabolic rate caused by your decreasing body weight. This, in turn, means that you burn more energy each and every minute of every day. All good news!

But the benefits don't stop there. Fit people *burn more fat*. So once you have lost weight, continuing to exercise makes your body a fat-burning machine that is much more effective at resisting weight gain. Furthermore, exercise and the amount of muscle you have affect your body's ability to respond to insulin—fit people need less insulin to maintain blood-glucose levels, because their muscles are primed and trained to respond quickly and effectively to incoming fuel. Alongside a healthy low-GI diet, these changes maximize your chances of maintaining a lean, fit body for life.

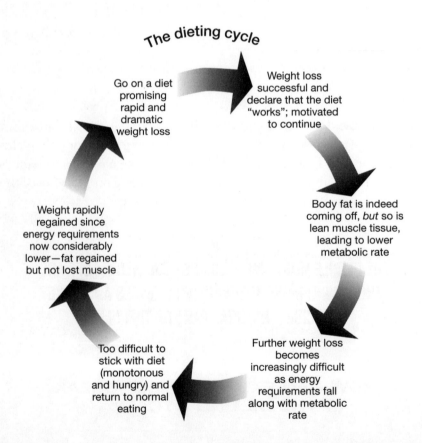

The dieting cycle

Go on a diet promising rapid and dramatic weight loss

Weight loss successful and declare that the diet "works"; motivated to continue

Body fat is indeed coming off, *but* so is lean muscle tissue, leading to lower metabolic rate

Further weight loss becomes increasingly difficult as energy requirements fall along with metabolic rate

Too difficult to stick with diet (monotonous and hungry) and return to normal eating

Weight rapidly regained since energy requirements now considerably lower—fat regained but not lost muscle

BEFORE YOU START THE ACTION PLAN

Remember, the Low GI Diet Revolution is not a fad diet. It is a serious diet and exercise program aimed at reducing body fat and *keeping it off for life*. Completing the Action Plan is the first step to better health and weight loss. It is followed by step two, Doing It for Life, which gives you the whole weight-loss *tool kit*—an assortment of strategies and tips to make lifestyle change easier, incorporating food, exercise, and behavioral change. The GI is just one of these tools, but it is an important one that makes a world of difference to your chances for successful long-term weight control.

Paul's story

I have tried every diet . . . and read every diet book. They never worked, and if I did lose weight, I put it back on with interest when I resumed normal eating habits. At 370 pounds I was desperate to find a way of eating that would work for me. My wife discovered *The New Glucose Revolution* . . . it was like someone had turned a light bulb on in my brain. Here was an eating plan that was a blueprint for life. Not a stunt diet, not a fad eating plan, but a commonsense approach to eating . . . that I believed I could stick with. Twelve months later I had lost 140 pounds, which was a direct consequence of eating the GI way and taking sensible exercise. My wife also lost 51 pounds over the same period. The GI way of eating has revolutionized my life and I have maintained exactly the weight loss since. I have never felt healthier and, more importantly, I never feel I am denying myself my choice of food . . . the GI way of eating is the best way to lose weight and maintain that loss. It saved my life.

Paul Jeffreys, *Diary of a Fat Man* (Penguin New Zealand 2003)

PART TWO

The 12-Week
Action Plan

About the Action Plan

In the 12-week Action Plan, we are going to start you on the road to freedom: freedom from the dieting nightmare and freedom from the burden of worrying about your weight.

Week by week, step by step, we will help you make good habits a natural part of your life. Each week we will ask you to focus on three goals—a food, exercise, and activity goal. You will begin by becoming more aware of your current eating patterns and behavior, which will help you to identify areas in which you could make changes for the better. We will also reveal a number of techniques for putting the seven dietary guidelines of the Low GI Diet Revolution into practice, so that healthy eating becomes a way of life.

At the same time, you will establish an exercise routine you can be proud of. You will be working on a combination of aerobic and resistance exercise that will increase your fat-burning muscle and tone your body.

Are you ready? This is it. It's time to take the first steps.

ABOUT THE MENU PLANS

For each week of the Action Plan, we have provided you with sample menus to give you ideas of what to eat on the road to better health. There is no need to follow these menus in a regimented fashion, but if you find it easier to do so, then feel free to. We have included lots of different foods throughout the menu plans to appeal to a broad range of tastes, but you can vary the menus according to your tastes using the simple guidelines to balanced low-GI meals found on pages 177–179.

How much food is right for you?

Everyone is different, so one eating plan will not work for everyone. Each one of us has different energy requirements, affected by such things as our size, how active we are, and even how much muscle we have. This is why diets of a set energy intake are not right for everyone. If you eat too little for your needs, you will find it hard to stick with the diet in the long term and you risk losing a greater proportion of muscle—which can set you on the yo-yo dieter's cycle of regaining the weight and getting fatter in the process. Your aim is to eat a *little* less than you need so that your body has to dig into those fat stores to make up the deficit.

For this reason, the sample menus do not give you quantities of foods, but are rather designed to illustrate appropriate food and meal choices to achieve a balanced low-GI diet. To give you an idea of recommended quantities of food, based on your current weight and gender, refer to the two tables that follow.

Step 1: Identify the energy level that corresponds to your current weight and gender.

Women		Men	
Weight (pounds)	**Energy level**	**Weight (pounds)**	**Energy level**
<154	1	<198	6
155–176	2	199–220	7
177–198	3	221–242	8
199–220	4	243–264	9
>220	5	>264	10

Step 2: Highlight the row that corresponds to your energy level—this gives you the recommended number of daily servings of each food type.

Recommended number of daily servings

Energy level	Carb-rich foods	Protein-rich foods	Fat-rich foods
1	3	3	2
2	4	4	2
3	5	5	3
4	6	6	3
5	7	7	3
6	8	8	4
7	9	9	4
8	10	10	4
9	11	11	5
10	12	12	5

In addition to the above servings, aim to eat at least five servings of vegetables and two servings of fruit every day.

Serving sizes

1 serving of vegetables

½ cup cooked vegetables (other than potato, sweet potato, or corn)

1 cup raw/salad vegetables

1 cup vegetable soup or juice

1 serving of fruit

1 medium piece or 2 small pieces (5 ounces) fresh fruit

1½ tablespoons raisins, 4–5 dried apricots/figs/prunes (1 ounce dried fruit)

½ cup fruit juice

1 cup diced or canned fruit

Carb-rich foods: 1 serving provides 20–30 grams carbohydrate

2 slices bread

1 cup breakfast cereal

½ cup oats or muesli

Serving sizes (continued)

½ cup cooked rice or other small grains such as cracked wheat (bulgur)

1 cup cooked pasta, noodles, or couscous

2 small potatoes or half a medium sweet potato (3½ ounces)

1 cup corn, beans, or chickpeas (can also count as a protein-rich food)

1 corn on the cob

Protein-rich foods: 1 serving provides 10–15 grams protein

1¾ ounces raw lean meat, poultry, fish, or seafood

3 slices (2 ounces) ham/pastrami/deli-sliced meat

1¾ ounces canned fish

1 cup skim milk

1 8-ounce carton low-fat yogurt

1 cup beans or chickpeas (can also count as a carb-rich food)

4 ounces tofu

2 eggs

Fat-rich foods: 1 serving provides 10 grams fat

2 teaspoons oil

1 tablespoon oil and vinegar dressing

2 teaspoons margarine/butter

3 teaspoons reduced-fat spread

3 teaspoons peanut butter*

1 ounce raw nuts or seeds*

2 tablespoons reduced-fat cream cheese*

2 ounces (2 pre-packaged slices) reduced-fat hard cheese*

1 ounce regular cheese*

*These foods are also good sources of protein, but have a particularly high fat content.

Example 1: Fiona's daily journal

Fiona currently weighs 167 pounds and is aiming to lose 13 pounds over the 12-week Action Plan. Using the above tables, she sees that she is on energy level 2 and should be aiming to eat four servings of carb-rich foods, four servings of protein-rich foods, and two servings of fat-rich foods in addition to at least five servings of vegetables and two of fruit every day.

A typical day for Fiona might look like this:

	Vegetables	Fruit	Carb-rich foods	Protein-rich foods	Fat-rich foods
Breakfast:					
½ cup muesli with ½ cup skim milk and a handful of sliced strawberries		1	1	½	
Lunch:					
1 cup of tomato soup with a sandwich of 2 slices whole-grain bread with 3 slices ham, 1 cup salad veggies, flavored with mustard	2		1	1	
Dinner:					
3½ ounces grilled salmon served with a cob of corn, ½ cup mixed-bean salsa, 2 cups green salad and 1 tablespoon olive oil and vinegar dressing	2		2	2	1
Snacks:					
1 cup fruit salad topped with ½ carton low-fat yogurt		1		½	
1 ounce almonds and 1 cup of vegetable juice	1			1	
TOTALS	5	2	4	4	2

Fiona's four servings of carbohydrate come from:
- ½ cup muesli (1 serving) at breakfast
- 2 slices bread (1) at lunchtime
- 1 corn on the cob (1) and ½ cup bean salsa (1) at dinner

Her four servings of protein come from:
- ½ cup skim milk (½) at breakfast
- 3 slices ham (1) at lunchtime
- 3½ ounces salmon (2) at dinner
- Half a carton yogurt (½) as a snack

Her two servings of fat come from:
- 1 tablespoon oil and vinegar dressing (1) at dinner
- 1 serving of nuts (1) as a snack

This day provides 1,296 calories, 79 grams of protein, 152 grams of carbohydrate, 40 grams of fat, and 31 grams of fiber.

Percent energy from the macronutrients

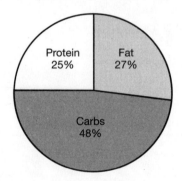

Example 2: Dave's daily journal

Fiona's husband, Dave, starts his program weighing 253 pounds. If Dave ate the same amount of food as Fiona, he would find himself ravenously hungry and would be unlikely to stick with the Action Plan for long. Using the tables, Dave sees that he is on energy level 9 and should be aiming for eleven servings each of carb- and protein-rich foods plus five servings of fat-rich foods in addition to at least five vegetable and two fruit servings every day.

Dave and Fiona want to be able to eat their meals together, and with the Action Plan they can—all Dave needs to do is change the quantities of food, sometimes adding foods, to be appropriate for his size and energy requirements.

A typical day for Dave might look like this:

	Vegetables	Fruit	Carb-rich foods	Protein-rich foods	Fat-rich foods
Breakfast:					
1 cup muesli with 1 cup skim milk and a handful of sliced strawberries		1	2	1	
2 boiled eggs with 2 slices grainy toast spread with 2 tablespoons butter/margarine			1	1	1
Lunch:					
1 cup tomato soup with 2 sandwiches of 4 slices whole-grain bread with 6 slices of ham, 2 cups salad veggies, flavored with mustard	3		2	2	
Dinner:					
7 ounces salmon grilled and served with a cob of corn, 1 cup mixed-bean salsa, 3 cups green salad and 2 tablespoons olive oil and vinegar dressing, plus 1 cup mashed sweet potato	3		4	4	2
Snacks:					
1 cup fruit salad topped with 1 carton low-fat yogurt		1		1	

	Vegetables	Fruit	Carb-rich foods	Protein-rich foods	Fat-rich foods
Snacks: 1 cup bean soup with 3 whole-grain crackers			2	1	
2 ounces almonds and a fruit smoothie made with 1 cup skim milk	1	1		1	2
TOTALS	7	3	11	11	5

Dave's typical day has similar proportions of energy from protein, fat, and carbohydrate, but larger quantities of each, providing 3,072 calories, 190 grams of protein, 100 grams of fat, 348 grams of carbohydrate, and 69 grams of fiber.

Percent energy from the macronutrients

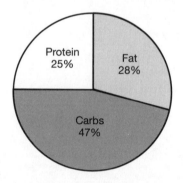

Of course, as you lose weight, you may find that you move down an energy level—this is because with less weight to move around, your energy requirements also fall. Reevaluate how much you should be eating every month to ensure the best success in reaching your goals.

While we suggest that most people start off by measuring their serving sizes according to the previous tables, some prefer a less structured approach. If this sounds like you, you may be able to use your appetite as the best indicator of how much food you need. To ensure that your meals are correctly balanced, follow these three simple steps when planning meals:

> **1.** *Start* with your low-GI carbohydrate.
>
> **2.** *Add* a generous serving of vegetables or fruit.
>
> **3.** *Plus* some protein for good measure, with a little healthy fat if you wish.

ABOUT THE EXERCISE PLANS

To gain the most benefit from the exercises outlined in the Action Plan, you need to work at an appropriate intensity—if the exercise feels too easy, you are not maximizing your energy expenditure or the amount of fat burned to fuel the exercise; if you try too hard, you will struggle to keep going for the allocated time, you will find it uncomfortable and unenjoyable, and you are unlikely to keep it up on a regular basis.

You don't need fancy equipment such as heart-rate monitors to measure your exercise intensity—all you need is a simple scale of how you feel. The Perceived Rate of Exertion (PRE) scale has been used for years by fitness instructors to guide their clients in their workouts. We will use a modified version of this scale to help you to maximize your fat loss and energy expenditure at each workout session. As you are exercising, ask yourself, on a scale of 1 to 10, how you are feeling, using the following table as a guide.

The PRE Scale

FOR HEALTH

1. At rest

2. Minimal exertion

3. Comfortable and could easily continue for some time

4. Starting to get a little breathless but relatively comfortable

FOR FITNESS

5. A little breathless and can feel heart rate elevated

6. Breathing harder, heart rate elevated but can still talk comfortably

7. Breathing hard, exercise much more difficult and cannot maintain for more than a few minutes

FOR PERFORMANCE

8. Much more intense and difficult to maintain, can keep going at this intensity for only a short time

9. Extremely intense exercise, cannot talk comfortably and breathing hard

10. Maximum intensity, which can be maintained for only a few seconds

The good news is that during the 12-week Action Plan, you will never be working above level 5. This means that you will never need to experience intense or uncomfortable exercise. Levels of intensity above 5 are useful for athletes who need to stretch their fitness levels to the extreme in order to improve their performance in their sport. Thankfully, if you are seeking the health benefits of exercise and aiming to lose body fat, working at the lower, more comfortable levels will better help you to reach your goals. In fact, in the early days of the program, you are going to be sticking to a PRE level of 3–4, the perfect level to improve your health and get you burning fat. As you progress and become fitter, we incorporate short sessions at level 5. This will help you to keep your weight under control for a lifetime as your body becomes a far more efficient fat-burning machine.

The exercise involved in the Action Plan incorporates both aerobic and resistance training:

- **Aerobic training** is any movement that gets you breathing a little harder—by definition, aerobic means "using oxygen." This sort of exercise works your heart and lungs and burns energy, helping you to increase your daily energy expenditure and burn body fat. We have opted to use walking as our aerobic exercise, but cycling, running, swimming, aerobics, rowing, and stepping are all also good forms of aerobic exercise.
- **Resistance training** is any exercise that makes your muscles work against a resistance. This includes lifting weights, using resistance bands, or simply using your own body weight as resistance. This sort of exercise is crucial to strengthen muscles, achieve and maintain good posture, and tone your body. In addition, by building a little more lean muscle mass, you increase your metabolic rate. As muscle is far more metabolically active than fat, the more muscle mass you have, the more energy you burn all of the time. To achieve fat loss and maintain that fat loss, resistance training offers great benefits and is an invaluable part of the Action Plan.

At the start of each week, get out your journal and schedule in a precise time for all of your walks and workouts. If you leave it to happen spontaneously, the week will be over before you know it and you won't even have started. Treat each exercise session as any other appointment and stick to it—if you have to postpone a session, make sure you reschedule it for another time. With the walking sessions, you have the option of breaking the walk into two shorter walks if you don't have enough time all at once. You could try doing ten minutes of walking first thing in the morning and the rest in the evening.

You won't need any special equipment. Simply wear comfortable, loose clothing and supportive walking shoes—sneakers are perfect, or use any comfortable, supportive shoe you have.

While it's commonly thought that moving quickly makes exercise harder, the opposite is in fact true for resistance exercise. To gain the best results from the resistance exercises, move slowly and focus on perfecting your technique. Try counting in seconds, taking two seconds to get to the end position and two seconds to get back to the start.

Remember that *anything* you do more than you are currently doing is a step in the right direction. Use the exercise plan as a guide and do as much as you can. If the weeks are progressing too quickly for you, simply stick with the same plan for a few more weeks, moving on to the next week's plan once you feel ready.

The resistance exercises may not be suitable for those with limiting injuries or conditions such as arthritis. If you feel pain at any time, you should stop the exercise and consult a qualified personal trainer for an individualized program.

WEEK 1

Are you ready to begin? For this first week, focus on the following goals:

▶ FOOD GOAL

Increase your awareness of what you eat and why.

▶ EXERCISE GOAL

Aim to walk at a steady, comfortable pace for a total of 20 minutes on four days. *Plus* complete the two resistance exercises outlined on three days.

▶ ACTIVITY GOAL

Rather than standing still on escalators and moving walkways, keep moving and walk to the end.

▶ FOOD FOR THOUGHT

What is the GI of your diet?

▶ FOOD GOAL

Increase your awareness of what you eat and why.

Your first dietary goal with the Action Plan is to keep a food journal to identify exactly what you usually eat and why you make the choices you do. You may think you already know what you eat, but there is nothing like writing it down to increase your awareness of all that you eat and drink.

Looking back over the record at the end of the week will enable you to compare your eating habits with the Low GI Diet Revolution's recommended food choices (see pages 37–52) and serving sizes (see pages 61–62), and help you identify foods that you could substitute or minimize. A food journal can also reveal links between what you eat and the mood, environment, or situations you find yourself in—we will look at alleviating problem areas next week.

- ▶ Choose a normal week in your life—one that is representative of most weeks (not one where you are away on vacation, for example).
- ▶ Use a small notebook that you can take everywhere and write down everything you eat and drink as soon as possible after you have eaten it (or while you are eating it). Note where you are, what you are doing, and how you feel.

You can also use the journal to write down your physical activity. We have included a template for your journal on page 289.

▶ EXERCISE GOAL

Aim to walk at a steady, comfortable pace for a total of 20 minutes on four days. *Plus* complete the two resistance exercises outlined on three days.

Walking

Using the PRE scale on page 67, aim to walk at about level 3—this means you should feel comfortable at all times and be able to carry on a conversation while walking. You should feel warmer as the blood flow around the body increases, taking fuel to your working muscles —this means you are burning more fat and increasing your daily energy expenditure.

Resistance Exercise

Lower-body exercises	Upper-body exercises	"Core" strength abdominals and back
Squats 2 sets of 10		Leg extensions 10 each leg

NEW EXERCISES

Squats

The squat is arguably the best lower-body exercise you can do. The muscles of your thighs and bottom are the biggest muscle group in the body, and this means exercises involving these muscles use the most energy—exactly what you want to help you lose body fat.

Strengthens and tones: thighs and bottom

How to do it:

1. Stand with your feet parallel and just wider than hip-distance apart. Extend your arms directly in front of you at chest height, with hands clasped.
2. Lengthen your spine by standing tall and pulling in your belly below the navel to support the lower back.
3. Imagine you have a chair behind you and sit back until you "touch" the imaginary chair. As you sit back, make sure you keep your arms parallel to the floor and your chest "proud."
4. Squeeze your bottom muscles and push your heels into the floor to get back to the standing position.

Remember: Throughout the exercise, keep your weight on the back two-thirds of your feet: you should be able to wiggle your toes. One last thing—don't forget to breathe normally.

How many: 2 sets of 10 with a short rest in between

Single-leg extensions

One of the most important groups of muscles for you to exercise is that involved in posture and back support. (These are the deep abdominal muscles that lie below the six-pack of stomach muscles you can see on the very lean men seen advertising unnecessary abdominal-trainer machines.) They lie across your body and act like a belt, holding in your waist to provide support, particularly for the lower back. By working this group of muscles you develop core strength that will immediately improve your posture (making you look slimmer), reduce the risk of back pain, and strengthen you from the inside out.

Strengthens and tones: the "core" (deep abdominals)

How to do it:

1. Lie flat on your back on the floor with your knees bent in toward your chest, and arms by your sides with hands flat to the floor.
2. Pull in your belly as if trying to shorten the distance between your navel and spine—it should feel as if you are bracing the abdominal wall. Extend one leg out parallel to the floor while keeping the abdominals braced.
3. Bring the leg back in and repeat on the other side.

Remember: Breathe normally (it's easy to hold your breath subconsciously during this exercise).
How many: 20 (10 on each leg)

Sample journal

Monday	Tuesday	Wednesday	Thursday	Friday	Saturday	Sunday
	20 min walk		20 min walk		20 min walk	20 min walk
	+ resistance exercises		+ resistance exercises		+ resistance exercises	
	25 min		25 min		25 min	20 min

▶ FOOD FOR THOUGHT
What is the GI of your diet?

Using the information from your food journal, answer the quiz below to gain a clearer idea of where you need to make changes to lower the GI of your diet.

What is the GI of your diet?

Simply circle the option that most closely matches your usual diet.

1. The type of bread I most often eat is

a. a whole-grain low-GI variety (see page 41 for examples)

b. sourdough or "health" bread

c. regular white or whole-grain sandwich bread

2. The type of breakfast cereal I usually eat is

a. traditional rolled oats, muesli, or a commercial low-GI type

b. a higher-fiber commercial cereal such as wheat biscuits or flakes

c. a low-fiber puffed or flaked cereal

3. I eat 2 or more different pieces of fruit

a. most days

b. 3–4 days a week

c. 1–2 days a week

4. I eat legumes (including baked beans, lentils, chickpeas, kidney beans, salad beans, etc.) or barley

a. 2 or more times a week

b. once a week

c. rarely or never

5. I eat pasta or noodles

a. 2 or more times a week

b. once a week

c. rarely or never

6. I eat sweet potato and or sweet corn as whole or partial substitutes for potato

a. 2 or more times a week

b. once a week

c. rarely or never

7. Of the following servings of food:

- 1 cup milk (any type)
- 1 cup yogurt (any type)
- ½ cup custard
- 2 scoops low-fat ice cream

I would eat at least 2 servings

a. most days

b. 3–4 days a week

c. 1–2 days a week or less

Your scorecard:

Score 1 point for each time you answered (a)

Score 2 points for each time you answered (b)

Score 3 points for each time you answered (c)

If your total is:

7–10 Well done—your diet is likely to have a low GI. The carbohydrate foods you have indicated you eat most frequently are low-GI choices. You may still need to consider serving sizes to facilitate weight loss. Keep reading, because there is lots more to a healthy low-GI diet than low-GI foods alone.

11–17 Your diet is likely to have an intermediate GI. This is true of the average diet of most people in Western countries. You have indicated that you eat a mixture of low-, medium-, and possibly high-GI carbohydrate choices, and, while variety is good, high-GI foods may be hindering your efforts at weight loss. Choosing more foods that fit option (a) will reduce the GI of your diet.

18–21 Your diet is likely to have a high GI. Many of your carbohydrate choices have high GI values, increasing your insulin demand and keeping your body in a state that favors fat storage. In order to lose weight, it will be beneficial to change at least half of your high-GI carb foods to those with a low GI. Choosing more foods that fit option (a) will reduce the GI of your diet.

WEEK 1 MENU PLAN

	BREAKFAST	SNACK
MONDAY	Whole-grain toast with peanut butter (no butter) and a glass of fruit or vegetable juice	Canned fruit snack pack
TUESDAY	Whole-grain toast with low-fat cheese	A banana
WEDNESDAY	Low-fat milk, coffee, or hot chocolate with raisin toast	Dried fruit and nut mix
THURSDAY	Natural muesli with low-fat milk, topped with fruit and fat-free yogurt	A banana
FRIDAY	High-fiber cereal with low-fat milk and fruit	An apple
SATURDAY	Sautéed mushrooms with parsley and shallots, low-GI toast, and a poached egg	A mandarin
SUNDAY	A boiled egg, lean bacon, tomato, and mushrooms, and a glass of vegetable juice	A small fruit smoothie

LUNCH	SNACK	DINNER
Sourdough rye with roast beef, horse-radish, sliced tomato, and snow pea sprouts	Reduced-fat ched-dar cheese with an apple and whole-grain crackers	Baked whitefish fillets with chopped parsley. Serve with chopped spinach and lemon, yellow squash, carrots, and a couple of baby new potatoes. Serve with low-fat yogurt.
Tuna, celery, onion, tomato, and olives tossed in balsamic vinaigrette with lettuce and whole-grain crackers	Low-fat yogurt	Vegetable Frittata (see page 232) and tossed salad. Baked apple and low-fat custard
Avocado, chicken, and lettuce wrap	Fresh fruit	Lean steak with mushrooms, sweet-potato mash, green beans, and zucchini
Salad with lettuce, celery, apple, wal-nuts, mayonnaise, and tuna	Low-fat ice cream in a cone	Tuna with canned tomatoes, artichoke quarters, kalamata olives, garlic, sliced zucchini, and tomato paste tossed with spiral pasta
Ramen noodle pork oriental soup	Low-fat yogurt	Pork and vegetable (broccoli, carrot, peppers, and onion) stir-fry with cashew nuts and basmati rice
Toasted soy-and-linseed English muffins spread with creamed corn, sliced fresh mushrooms, and a sprinkle of grated cheese, heated under the grill	Oatmeal cookies	Lamb roast with mint sauce, baked sweet potato, pumpkin, onion, and steamed peas, beans, and cauliflower; fresh fruit salad
Thai beef salad made with lean beef strips, mixed salad greens, and a dressing of chili, garlic, lime juice, brown sugar, and Thai fish sauce, sprinkled with cellophane noodles	A small handful of almonds	Minestrone soup; low-fat yogurt and fruit

WEEK 2

Being overweight is *not* about lacking willpower, and if you have ever been on a diet, you will know that to be true. Changing habits that are ingrained in our daily lives is extremely difficult and takes time (about a year, to be exact!). In Week 1, the focus was on becoming more aware of what you eat and starting to incorporate more low-GI foods into your diet. This week, we help you pinpoint your bad habits and set goals that will lead you toward healthier habits. Your goals to work on this week are:

▶ FOOD GOAL
Pinpoint your bad habits and set three SMART food goals.

▶ EXERCISE GOAL
Aim to walk at a steady, comfortable pace for 20 minutes on four days. *Plus* complete the three resistance exercises outlined on three days.

▶ ACTIVITY GOAL
For all short journeys that would take less than five minutes in the car, walk instead.

▶ FOOD FOR THOUGHT
Time for a change.

▶ FOOD GOAL

Pinpoint your bad habits and set three SMART food goals.

Having put in the effort and recorded your eating patterns last week, you now have the opportunity to identify the eating habits that you're going to change. Making changes begins with setting goals. Ideally, your goals should be **S**pecific, **M**easurable, **A**chievable, **R**ealistic, and **T**ime-specific (SMART).

For example, it is unrealistic to set the goal "I'll stop eating chocolate" and may be unachievable to say "I will bring my lunch from home every day." These all-or-nothing goals tend to set us up for failure and are not helpful in achieving long-term changes.

Examples of SMART goals in these instances:

- ▶ I will allow myself a chocolate bar once a month.
- ▶ I will start preparing my own lunch to take to work on Mondays and Tuesdays.

Habits that you want to change may also relate to your eating behavior. The following checklist will help you identify problem eating behaviors. Referring back to your food journal if you need to, check off any of the following that are regular events for you.

- ❏ I eat too many snacks
- ❏ I eat irregular meals
- ❏ I nibble all day
- ❏ I eat while watching television
- ❏ I eat when preparing food
- ❏ I serve or am served more than I need, but eat it anyway
- ❏ I impulse-buy unplanned foods
- ❏ I eat when I'm not hungry, but because I'm bored, tired, depressed, or angry
- ❏ I eat out too often
- ❏ I eat while driving or traveling
- ❏ I eat too fast
- ❏ I linger at the table, eating more even though I'm satisfied

❑ I go back for seconds

❑ I overeat night snacks

❑ I always finish my plate even if I feel full

❑ I drink too much alcohol

❑ I buy foods for the family that I don't intend to eat but can't resist

Now, given your checklist of problem eating behaviors and your food journal, select two or three of your eating habits or food choices that you would like to change and brainstorm possible solutions.

Set yourself three goals relating to what or how you eat. Remember, your goals must be relevant to you and your situation and should be specific, measurable, achievable, realistic, and time-specific. Commit to these goals, trying to adhere to them as much as you can. At the end of the week, think about how successful you were in sticking to your goals. Did they work for you? Are you willing to keep them going? If the answer is no, then try setting different goals, based on different solutions to your habits, and keep experimenting until you find the change that works for you.

▶ EXERCISE GOAL

Aim to walk at a steady, comfortable pace for 20 minutes on four days. *Plus* complete the three resistance exercises outlined on three days.

Resistance exercises

Lower-body exercises	Upper-body exercises	"Core" strength abdominals and back
Squats 2 sets of 10	Assisted push-ups 2 sets of 10	Leg extensions 10 each leg

NEW EXERCISE

Assisted push-ups

The push-up is undeniably one of the best upper-body exercises you can do. The push-up involves the muscles of the chest, shoulders, and arms and is therefore an efficient means of toning the upper body all at once.

Why do most people hate push-ups? The answer is easy—because they are hard! In fact, they are even harder if you are carrying too much body weight, since you are essentially lifting your own body weight against gravity. Here is a modified version of the traditional push-up, which enables you to gain the benefits of the exercise but makes it easier for you to perform it correctly. You will need a low coffee table—alternatively, use the second or third bottom step of your stairs.

Strengthens and tones: chest, shoulders, and arms

How to do it:
1. Start in a kneeling position with your hands wider than your shoulders on the edge of the table/stair. Move your knees back until your body is a straight diagonal line from head to knee.
2. Slowly lower your chest toward the edge of the table/stair while keeping your back flat and without letting your bottom stick up.
3. At the bottom of the move, your elbows should be directly above your hands—adjust your hand position as appropriate before returning slowly to the starting position.

How many: 2 sets of 10 repetitions with a short rest in between

Sample journal

Monday	Tuesday	Wednesday	Thursday	Friday	Saturday	Sunday
	20 min walk		20 min walk		20 min walk	20 min walk
	+ resistance exercises		+ resistance exercises		+ resistance exercises	
	25 min		25 min		25 min	20 min

▶ FOOD FOR THOUGHT
Time for a change.

The fact that you are reading this page suggests that you are at least *contemplating* making some changes to the way you eat. People don't make changes instantaneously; they work their way up to it gradually, often going through definable stages. A description of the stages of change in relation to our eating habits looks like this:

Pre-contemplation

At this stage you're not thinking about changing your eating habits; what you're doing is appropriate for *you* at this time in your life. You could read this book and then put it away for later reference.

Contemplation

Now you're beginning to think about change, but just haven't got around to it. Weigh the benefits and costs of making a change. If the benefits outweigh the costs, then you're ready to move on to preparation.

Preparation

Now you have decided to change and are preparing to do so. Attempting change without prior planning makes relapse more likely. So ask yourself, what do you think you *can* change?

Action

You are now actually in the process of making changes to the way you eat. Your goals ought to be SMART—**S**pecific, **M**easurable, **A**chievable, **R**ealistic, and **T**ime-specific. For example:

- Every two days, buy four nice pieces of fresh fruit to eat.
- Buy and use only fat-reduced milk for the next month as a trial.

Your goals must be relevant to you and your situation, so checking back through your food journal could be a good place from which to start planning your behavior changes.

Maintenance

At this point, you're committed to maintaining your changes and have no desire to return to your old ways. You face relapses every so often, but getting through them will lead to your changes becoming your new healthy habits.

Identifying your current stage of change should help you move forward to the next stage.

At what stage of change are you?

Circle the answer that best fits you and identify your current stage using the key below.

Have you been trying to lose weight?

a. Yes, I have been working on losing weight for at least three months.

b. Yes, I have been trying to lose weight within the last three months.

c. No, but I intend to start now.

d. No, and I do not intend to at the moment.

Key:

Answer (a) = maintenance stage

Answer (b) = action stage

Answer (c) = contemplation/preparation stage

Answer (d) = pre-contemplation stage

A word of warning: change can be difficult, and changing the way you eat is no exception. Even with all the willpower in the world, celebrations, cheesecakes, cravings, nights out, or chocolate will always be lurking around the corner, waiting to test your resolve. It might help to bear in mind that normal, healthy eating includes all foods, and "lapses" are just a normal part of change.

Our tips for approaching dietary change

1. Aim to make changes gradually. Acknowledge your stage of change.

2. Attempt the easiest changes first. Nothing inspires like success!

3. Break big changes into a number of smaller changes.

4. Accept lapses in your habits as a characteristic of being human.

If you feel like you need some extra help in changing the way you eat, seek out professional assistance from a registered dietitian (RD). (For details on finding an RD near you, see page 216.)

WEEK 2 MENU PLAN

	BREAKFAST	SNACK
MONDAY	Fruit bread lightly spread with ricotta cheese and jam	An apple and a few almonds
TUESDAY	Multigrain English muffin with scrambled egg and tomato juice	2 kiwi fruit
WEDNESDAY	Whole-grain toast with hazelnut spread and an apple	A small handful of unsalted nuts
THURSDAY	Low-fat vanilla yogurt with sliced fresh nectarine and strawberries, topped with muesli	An Apricot and Almond Cookie (see page 259)
FRIDAY	Low-GI cereal topped with sliced pears and low-fat milk, and freshly squeezed orange juice	2 ginger nut cookies
SATURDAY	Lean grilled bacon with sliced tomato on whole-grain toast	A low-fat fruit yogurt
SUNDAY	Oatmeal with a garnish of frozen or fresh berries, low-fat natural yogurt, and a sprinkle of brown sugar	A slice of raisin toast

LUNCH	SNACK	DINNER
Ham and salad on whole-grain roll, skim-milk latte	Wedge of melon	Moroccan-style Lentil and Vegetable Stew with Couscous (see page 254)
Greek salad with low-fat feta and olives and a small whole-grain roll	Some low-fat ice cream	Tandoori chicken with basmati rice, lentil dal, and cucumber *raita* plus a mango chutney
Toasted sourdough with avocado, sliced tomato, and grilled lean bacon or double-smoked ham	Fresh orange quarters	Lamb shish kebabs with garlic and tahini sauce served with tabbouleh and pieces of pita bread
Garden salad with sliced chicken breast	A fresh pear	Spinach and ricotta cannelloni with pine nuts and tomato sauce; serve with a mixed green salad with vinaigrette
Whole-grain bread with shaved ham, grated carrot, shredded lettuce, sliced tomato, low-fat grated cheese, and mayonnaise	Fruit salad	Cook a whole fish, such as snapper, by wrapping in two layers of foil and setting on the barbecue for 25–30 minutes; serve with roasted sweet-potato wedges
Tuna, onion, lettuce, and cheese on a whole-grain roll	Fruit and nut mix	Shrimp and Mango Salad with Chili-Lime Dressing (see page 247); a wedge of melon with a scoop of low-fat ice cream
Tacos topped with refried beans, diced tomato, shredded lettuce, avocado, and grated reduced-fat cheese	An apple	Barbecued steak with roasted-vegetable salad and green salad

WEEK 3

Unless you have diabetes and are diligent about testing your blood-glucose levels, you are probably completely unaware of your own fluctuations over the course of a day. Yet these fluctuations can have a major effect on what, how much, and when you eat, as well as determine whether you store or burn body fat. This week, focus on these goals:

▶ FOOD GOAL

Minimize your blood-glucose fluctuations by getting the smart carbs going.

▶ EXERCISE GOAL

Aim to walk at a steady, comfortable pace (level 3 on the PRE scale) for a total of 20 minutes on five days. *Plus* complete the four resistance exercises on three days.

▶ ACTIVITY GOAL

Arrange a social activity for the weekend that does not involve food or drink, but something active instead. Why not try going to the golf course, cycling in the park, or bowling with a bunch of friends?

▶ FOOD FOR THOUGHT

Why your blood-glucose level is so important.

▶ FOOD GOAL

Minimize your blood-glucose fluctuations by getting the right carbs going.

Want to keep your engine running smoothly all day? Then *slow release* low-GI carbs are the ones for you. The slow digestion rate of low-GI carbs trickles fuel into your system at a steady rate, reducing insulin levels and minimizing blood-glucose fluctuations. This small change can potentially make a huge difference to your waistline in the long term. It's the starchy carb staples in your diet that have the greatest impact—so check to make sure you are eating the right carbs by using the following table.

Starchy staples	Minimize these high-GI choices	Use these low-GI varieties instead
The bread you eat	Soft white bread	Sourdough
	Light and airy, smooth-textured white and whole-grain bread	Dense whole-grain breads
	Scones, fruit, nut bread	Fruit bread
The cereals in your pantry	Refined, commercial processed cereals	Traditional rolled oats and barley-based cereals
Main-meal carbs	Potatoes: mashed, chips, and french fries	Sweet potato, sweet corn, pasta, noodles, butter beans, lentils, chickpeas
	Jasmine, brown, and arborio rice	Basmati or koshihikari (sushi) rice
The foods you snack on	Light and crispy crackers, doughnuts, pretzels	Fresh or dried fruit, low-fat yogurt, nuts

Base your food goals this week around making your starchy staples the smart low-GI types.

▶ EXERCISE GOAL

Aim to walk at a steady, comfortable pace (level 3 on the PRE scale) for a total of 20 minutes on five days. *Plus* complete the four resistance exercises on three days.

Resistance exercises

Lower-body exercises	Upper-body exercises	"Core" strength abdominals and back
Squats 2 sets of 10	Assisted push-ups 2 sets of 10	Leg extensions 10 each leg
Lunges 10 each leg		

NEW EXERCISE

Lunges

This week we add one more exercise for the lower body. Lunges are a little more difficult than squats, because one leg has to work harder than the other. They are very effective at working the thighs and bottom, with the lower leg also doing some work for a complete lower-body workout. The most common mistake is to have your feet too close together, which makes it difficult to lunge without bringing your weight forward over the front foot—aim for a long stride and work on keeping the upper body upright, with your chest proud. Use a broom handle or the back of a chair to help with balance when you first do this exercise; as you become stronger you will be able to do it without assistance.

Strengthens: bottom and legs

How to do it:
1. Stand with your feet hip-width apart and then step one foot back in a long stride behind you. Your feet should still be parallel —you should not feel like you are tightrope walking, but are in a strong, tall stance.
2. Center your body weight between your feet and tuck your hips underneath to maintain a long, strong spine. Slowly drop your body weight down until your front thigh is parallel to the floor and the back knee is under your hip.
3. Push your front heel into the floor to push you back to the top.

Remember: Your back heel should not touch the floor during the exercise —you should be up on the ball of your foot throughout the motion.

How many: 10 lunges on each leg

Sample journal

Monday	Tuesday	Wednesday	Thursday	Friday	Saturday	Sunday
20 min walk	20 min walk		20 min walk		20 min walk	20 min walk
	+ resistance exercises		+ resistance exercises		+ resistance exercises	
20 min	30 min		30 min		30 min	20 min

▶ FOOD FOR THOUGHT
Why your blood-glucose level is so important.

A normal blood-glucose level is the difference between life and death—literally. A low blood-glucose level can result in coma and death within minutes. A high blood-glucose level will kill you, too, but the process takes years. If a high blood-glucose condition is not treated, it will result in blindness, heart disease, and kidney failure. Unless you have diabetes or prediabetes, such morbid thoughts won't trouble you. In healthy individuals, blood-glucose levels are held automatically within a fairly narrow range (between 70–110 mg/dL). They go up and down when we eat; if we skip a meal (or exclude carbs), the liver draws on its reserves of carbohydrates. When those run out, the liver will make glucose using building blocks from the breakdown of protein and fat stores. The reason for such fine control is that glucose is virtually the sole fuel of our metabolically expensive brain. Without glucose, it shuts down and everything else grinds to a halt, too.

One in four adults (especially those with excess fat around the middle) has undesirably high blood-glucose levels. Every time they eat, their blood glucose increases rapidly and stays high for the following two to three hours. During that time, excess glucose circulates to all the tissues and organs around the body. The cells lining the blood vessels and those in the eyes and kidneys are extremely vulnerable because they can't control the amount of glucose that enters them. The end result is oxidative stress caused by highly reactive oxygen molecules. These "free radicals" inflame cells, eventually causing swelling, scarring, thickening, hardening, and the inability to dilate and contract as needed. In time, the chances of a small blood clot lodging and blocking a narrow artery increase. If it happens in a major vessel of the heart, you have a heart attack on your hands. If it's a minor vessel in the heart, it causes chest pain (angina). If it happens in the brain, it's called a stroke.

But that's not all: high blood-glucose levels affect the function of many proteins and enzymes, such that the chances of dying prematurely from any cause are higher. You don't need to be in the diabetic range to be at risk. High glucose and insulin levels fuel the growth of abnormal cells that cause various types of cancer—including breast, colon, endometrial, and pancreatic.

High glucose levels also spell trouble for weight control, because insulin will be secreted in an effort to bring the glucose level down. High insulin in turn causes insulin resistance, causing even higher insulin levels—a vicious cycle. Insulin drives glucose into the "engines" in each cell, forcing them to burn glucose and pushing fat to the side. In time, fat accumulates all around the body—in the blood (causing high triglycerides), in the liver (causing fatty liver), and in the abdomen (causing the most dangerous form of excess body fat).

Rapid rises and falls in blood glucose are also blamed for increasing appetite. The suddenly low glucose level stimulates the release of stress hormones such as cortisol, which stimulate hunger, causing you to think about the next meal. Studies show that slowly digested and absorbed low-GI carbs induce greater satiety, delaying the time to the next meal and/or reducing energy intake in comparison to their quickly digested counterparts.

WEEK 3 MENU PLAN

	BREAKFAST	SNACK
MONDAY	Natural muesli with low-fat yogurt and peach slices	Whole-wheat crackers and low-fat sliced cheese
TUESDAY	Multigrain English-muffin melts: top with creamed corn, sliced mushrooms, and low-fat mozzarella	2 kiwi fruit or mandarins
WEDNESDAY	Whole-grain toast spread with your favorite nut butter, plus a bowl of fresh chopped melon	Fresh carrot and pineapple juice
THURSDAY	Fruit and nut bar and a skim-milk cappuccino	A handful of cherries or other small fruit
FRIDAY	Egg flip made with low-fat milk, whole egg, vanilla, and sugar	An apple
SATURDAY	Sweet-corn fritters with fried tomato and onion	A bunch of grapes
SUNDAY	Sautéed mushrooms with parsley and shallots on low-GI toast with a poached egg	A small banana

LUNCH	SNACK	DINNER
Pasta salad with canned corn, peas, diced red pepper, grated carrot, chopped tomato, and mayonnaise	Small handful of almonds	Pan-fry a lean steak, then deglaze pan by adding a little red wine, beef stock, and 1 teaspoon Dijon mustard. Simmer for a minute, then pour over steaks. Serve with steamed or microwaved new potatoes and broccoli.
Flat bread with hummus, tabbouleh salad, and falafel	Low-fat banana smoothie	Dust boneless fish fillets (e.g., ocean perch) in corn flour. Melt 1 teaspoon margarine in a frying pan and add the juice of an orange and a lemon. Add the fish, cover and poach until starting to flake, turning once. Serve with steamed vegetables.
Canned tuna with lettuce, tomato, cucumber, feta, olives, and balsamic dressing with a whole-grain roll	A bunch of grapes	Eggplant and Zucchini Pilaf with Lamb (see pages 244–245), plus a low-fat fruit yogurt
Sweet-potato salad: grilled red pepper with steamed sweet potato and salad greens in balsamic dressing	Whole-grain toast and chocolate hazelnut spread	Tomato-and-onion omelet with green salad, plus sliced pineapple and low-fat ice cream
Cheese, tomato, lettuce, beets, and grated carrot on a whole-grain sandwich	Low-fat yogurt	Chicken and Rice Salad (see page 239)
Stir-fry Asian mixed vegetables with cubed firm tofu and garlic, ginger, soy sauce and honey, stirred with Hokkien noodles	A handful of popcorn and a small orange juice	Rosemary-studded rack of lamb with sweet-potato mash, green beans, and slow-roasted tomatoes, plus a low-fat chocolate mousse
Salmon frittata with tomato onion salsa, salad greens, and a slice of sourdough bread	Fruit with a scoop of low-fat ice cream	Vegetarian (bean) nachos made with salt-reduced oven-baked corn chips, served with avocado salsa

WEEK 4

You are four weeks into the Action Plan now, so it is a good time to reevaluate your food quantities based on your current weight, using the tables on page 60–61.

Focus on the following goals this week:

▶ FOOD GOAL

Lowering the GI of your diet by eating fewer processed foods.

▶ EXERCISE GOAL

Aim to walk at a slightly more brisk but still comfortable pace (level 4 on the PRE scale), for a total of 20 minutes on five days. *Plus* try to complete each of the two resistance workouts, focusing on the upper and lower body respectively, twice during the week.

▶ ACTIVITY GOAL

Whenever you are talking on the telephone, stand up, pace the floor, and stretch.

▶ FOOD FOR THOUGHT

How and why foods vary in their GI values.

▶ FOOD GOAL

Lowering the GI of your diet by eating fewer processed foods.

Oatmeal, barley, split peas, and lentils are remnants from our grand-parents' generation that once served us so well. Today we recognize these as some of the lowest-GI foods—high in fiber, rich in nutrients, bulky and filling—it is a shame they dwindled in popularity. Once, a hearty bowl of porridge was enough to sustain a person throughout the morning; now, many people rely on a quick bowl of crispy light flakes. This highly processed alternative is digested so quickly that it spikes blood glucose and insulin levels and leaves you hungry by mid-morning.

This week, consider how many processed foods you rely on and come up with alternatives. Wise ways to lower the GI of your diet include:

- ▶ Choose fewer processed starchy foods—use old-fashioned rolled oats, pearl barley, lentils, split peas, and chickpeas. Limit your intake of commercial crackers, cookies, and cakes.
- ▶ Look for low-GI snacks such as low-fat yogurts, fresh fruit, dried fruit and nut mix, and low-fat milk.
- ▶ Combine high-GI with low-GI foods to produce an interme-diate overall GI—lentils plus rice, tabbouleh plus bread, and potato mixed with sweet potato.
- ▶ Add a little acid to your meal—vinaigrette with salad, yogurt with cereal, lemon juice on vegetables, sourdough bread. All of these foods contain acids, which slow stomach emptying and lower your blood-glucose response to the carbohydrate with which they are eaten.

■

AIM FOR AT LEAST ONE LOW-GI CARB PER MEAL.

■

▶ **EXERCISE GOAL**

Aim to walk at a slightly more brisk but still comfortable pace (level 4 on the PRE scale), for a total of 20 minutes on five days. *Plus* try to complete each of the two resistance workouts, focusing on the upper and lower body respectively, twice during the week.

Resistance exercises

We have now split the resistance training into two workouts. The first focuses on the lower body and the second on the upper body. The "core" abdominals and back are worked in each one, as these areas are so important for your posture and strength.

Workout 1	Lower-body exercises	"Core" strength abdominals and back
	Squats 2 sets of 10	Three-quarter hover 2 x 20 seconds
	Lunges 10 each leg	
Workout 2	**Upper-body exercises**	
	Assisted push-ups 2 sets of 10	Leg extensions 10 each leg
	Standing tricep extensions 2 sets of 10	

NEW EXERCISES

Three-quarter hover

This exercise is fantastic for developing core strength and narrowing your waist. It may feel challenging to start with, but you will be amazed at how quickly you improve and reap the rewards of your efforts.

Strengthens and tones: waist

How to do it:

1. Lie face-down on the floor with your toes turned under and prop yourself up on your elbows.
2. Now lift your hips until they are in line with your shoulders and feet—it's important to make sure you don't stick your bottom out but maintain a straight line through the body from shoulder to knee.

3. As you hold the position, think of narrowing your waist and breathe normally.

How long: Hold the hover position for 20 seconds, rest for a few moments, and then repeat for a further 20 seconds.

Standing tricep extensions

The back of the upper arms is a common problem area for women in particular—we tend to store body fat here and lack muscle tone. You will need a weight to provide resistance in this exercise. You can buy small hand-held weights at any good sports shop or department store. Alternatively, improvise from your kitchen cupboard: a bag of rice or an unopened can may be used as a good starting weight—anything around the one-pound mark.

Strengthens and tones: the back of the upper arm

How to do it:
1. Stand tall and hold the weight overhead with both hands, with your arms straight. Make sure you are standing with good posture and eyes straight ahead rather than looking up at the weight.
2. Keeping your arms close to your ears, lower the weight behind your head.
3. Keeping the upper arm still, lift the weight back to the top.

How many: 2 sets of 10 with a short rest between sets

Sample journal

Monday	Tuesday	Wednesday	Thursday	Friday	Saturday	Sunday
20 min walk	20 min walk		20 min walk		20 min walk	20 min walk
+ workout 1	+ workout 2		+ workout 1		+ workout 2	
25 min	25 min		25 min		25 min	20 min

▶ FOOD FOR THOUGHT
How and why foods vary in their GI values.

From a weight-loss point of view, the longer the process of digestion takes and the more gradual the rise and fall in blood glucose, the better.

You don't have to eat all of your carbs in low-GI forms. Studies have shown that when a low- and a high-GI food are combined in one meal (such as lentils and rice), the overall blood-glucose response is intermediate between the two. You can keep both glucose and insulin levels lower over the course of the whole day if you choose at least one low-GI food at each meal.

What determines a food's GI value?

The speed with which carbs reach the bloodstream has little to do with sugar or fiber content. In fact, many sugary foods produce lower blood-glucose responses—gram for gram of carbohydrate—than many whole-meal products. By far the most important factor is the physical state of the starch in a food. If the starch granules have swollen and burst, that food will be digested in a flash. On the other hand, if they are still present in their "native" state, as found in raw food, then the process of digestion will take much longer. Advances in food processing over the past one hundred years have had a profound effect on the overall GI values of the carbohydrates we eat.

How do we know if a food is low-GI?

The only sure way of knowing the GI value of a food is by measuring it. This means having a group of volunteers eat the food in a controlled setting and comparing their blood-glucose levels after the food with their levels after the same carbohydrate load of a standard food, such as glucose. It is a lengthy and labor-intensive procedure, but at least 1,500 foods have already been tested, and more are being tested all the time in laboratories around the world.

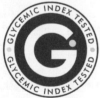 Watch out for this symbol on foods! It is your guarantee that the GI value on the label is correct (it has been tested by an accredited laboratory). This will also assure you that the food makes a nutritious contribution to your diet. Visit the Web site for more details: www.gisymbol.com.au.

Factors that influence the GI value of a food

Carbohydrate

Remember, only carbohydrate foods have GI values. So any food that is high in carbohydrate has a measurable GI value, but you can't guess what it is without testing it by the standard procedure. If the carbo-hydrate is predominantly in the form of starch, particularly cooked starch, the food is likely to have a high GI.

Example: cooked flour products such as bread, pancakes, and doughnuts

Fat
Fat tends to slow down stomach emptying, so high-fat foods often have lower GI values. This doesn't necessarily make high-fat foods good for you.

Example: potato chips, french fries

Protein
If your carbohydrate food is also high in protein, its GI value may be lower thanks to slower digestion or a higher insulin response.

Example: Kellogg's Special K

Acidity
Just like fat, acid tends to slow down stomach emptying and lowers the GI value of carbohydrate foods with which it is eaten. Sometimes the food itself is acidic by nature.

Example: vinaigrette on salad with bread

Soluble fiber
Although you can't see soluble fiber in food, the way it increases the viscosity of your intestinal contents will slow down carbohydrate digestion and lower the GI value.

Example: old-fashioned rolled oats

Is it as nature intended?
The less processed the food, the more likely it is to have a low GI value. The intact seed coat around whole grains contributes to their low GI value.

Example: legumes

Sugar
Just because a food is sweet, it isn't necessarily high-GI. The GI value depends on the type of sugar and the other sources of carbohydrate in the food. Table sugar or sucrose has an intermediate GI value.

WEEK 4 MENU PLAN

	BREAKFAST	SNACK
MONDAY	Old-fashioned rolled oats	A handful of peanuts in the shell
TUESDAY	Half a grapefruit followed by boiled eggs with sourdough toast	An orange
WEDNESDAY	Natural muesli with sliced apple, low-fat milk, and natural yogurt	A handful of dried apricots
THURSDAY	Fruit salad with low-fat natural yogurt and a sprinkle of mixed nuts and seeds	Low-fat flavored milk
FRIDAY	Old-fashioned oatmeal topped with fresh or frozen raspberries and low-fat natural yogurt	Low-fat fruit yogurt
SATURDAY	Poached eggs with wilted spinach, grilled tomato, and dry-fried mushrooms with a slice of whole-grain bread	A cup of vegetable soup
SUNDAY	Heavy fruit toast with low-fat cream cheese and finely sliced apple or pear	A handful of cherries

LUNCH	SNACK	DINNER
Bowl of minestrone soup with whole-grain bread dipped in a teaspoon of olive oil	A pear	Grilled lean lamb fillets sliced and served on a sweet potato salad and topped with a spoonful of chutney
Mixed box of sushi with miso soup	Small handful of dried fruit and nut mix	Grilled salmon fillet with mashed sweet potato and steamed broccoli, green beans, and carrots
Bowl of bean soup with a slice of toasted whole-grain bread	Slice of multigrain toast with a teaspoon of peanut butter	Cover a skinless chicken breast with a basic tomato sauce (ready-made pasta sauce is fine) and bake for 30 minutes. Serve with a steamed ear of corn, wilted spinach, and dry-fried mushrooms.
A whole-wheat pita bread filled with hummus, tabbouleh, lettuce, and sliced tomato	Fresh fruit	Chili con carne made with lean beef and kidney beans, served with steamed basmati rice and a large green salad
Steak sandwich—grilled minute steak in multigrain bread with lettuce, beets, grated carrot, tomato, and mustard	Carrot sticks with hummus dip	Bake a firm whitefish fillet in white wine, lemon juice, chopped ginger, garlic, and coriander for 20 minutes. Serve with steamed sushi rice and stir-fried Asian greens in oyster sauce.
Lentil soup with whole-grain bread and low-fat cheese	Strawberries topped with natural yogurt and some flaked toasted almonds	Grill a chicken breast, slice and serve over a small bowl of pasta in tomato sauce accompanied by a large green salad.
Tuna salad with shallots, baby beets, olives, cherry tomatoes, cucumber, blanched green beans, and peppers, drizzled with a little olive oil and balsamic vinegar dressing	Muesli and Honey Slice (see page 260)	Grilled or barbecued pork skewers marinated in spicy sauce, served with a large mixed salad and a few baby new potatoes

WEEK 5

We have already learned that low-GI foods keep us full longer, and this week we now focus on how protein-rich foods can also help. Focus on the following goals this week:

▶ FOOD GOAL
Incorporate a lean protein source in every meal.

▶ EXERCISE GOAL
Aim to walk at the same pace as last week (level 4 on the PRE scale) for a total of 20 minutes on six days. *Plus* try to complete each of the two resistance workouts, focusing on the upper and lower body respectively, three times during the week.

▶ ACTIVITY GOAL
Whenever there is the option of taking the stairs, the elevator, or an escalator, choose to take the stairs for at least one flight. If you are heading for the 12th floor of a building, for example, take the stairs to the 1st floor before taking the elevator the rest of the way.

▶ FOOD FOR THOUGHT
The real deal on protein and health.

▶ FOOD GOAL

Incorporate a lean protein source in every meal.

Clearly the best foods for weight control are those that fill you up and keep you from getting hungry again too quickly. Protein-rich foods tend to be the most satiating, followed by carbohydrate-rich and, in last place, fat-rich foods. In practical terms, this means that by including a protein-rich food in each meal, you can help to satisfy your appetite and delay the return of hunger, seeing you through to the next meal or snack.

While it is unlikely that you have been eating insufficient protein to meet your body's needs, if you have been focusing on reducing your fat intake, you may have inadvertently made it difficult for yourself by not taking advantage of the power of protein-rich foods to fill you up. A typical dieters' lunch of a salad, sandwich, or bowl of vegetable soup may sound like a healthy choice, but on their own these meals are likely to leave you ravenous within a couple of hours of eating them, particularly if the meal included high-GI carbs such as white bread. Add a protein-rich food to the meal, along with a moderate portion of a low-GI carb, and you have a more balanced and filling meal.

For example:

▶ At breakfast, include low-fat milk, yogurt, eggs, lean bacon, smoked salmon, sardines, cottage cheese, ricotta cheese, herrings, nuts, or nut butters.
▶ At light and main meals, include lean meat, poultry, fish, reduced-fat cheese, eggs, tofu, or legumes (beans or lentils).

▶ EXERCISE GOAL

Aim to walk at the same pace as last week (level 4 on the PRE scale) for a total of 20 minutes on six days. *Plus* try to complete each of the two resistance workouts, focusing on the upper and lower body respectively, three times during the week.

Resistance exercises

Workout 1	Lower-body exercises	"Core" strength abdominals and back
	Squats 2 sets of 10	Three-quarter hover 2 x 20 seconds
	Lunges 10 each leg	Pointer 10 each side
Workout 2	**Upper-body exercises**	
	Assisted push-ups 2 sets of 10	Leg extensions 10 each leg
	Standing tricep extensions 2 sets of 10	

NEW EXERCISE

Pointer

This is a simple but effective exercise for strengthening the back and bottom muscles, as well as continuing to work on your core abdominal strength.

Strengthens and tones: back, bottom, and core abdominals

How to do it:

1. Start on all fours and align your spine by keeping your eyes on the floor just in front of your hands and pulling your navel up toward your spine, without allowing your back to arch. Your hands and your knees should be hip- and shoulder-width apart.
2. Lift your right hand and left leg and extend slowly over a count of four until they are straight and in line with your torso—you are aiming for length rather than height. Hold for 4 seconds before slowly pulling the arm and leg back in close to the torso, then repeat the movement.

3. Repeat with the left arm and the right leg.

How many: Repeat 10 extensions on each side

Sample journal

Monday	Tuesday	Wednesday	Thursday	Friday	Saturday	Sunday
20 min walk	20 min walk	20 min walk	20 min walk		20 min walk	20 min walk
+ workout 1	+ workout 2	+ workout 1	+ workout 2		+ workout 1	+ workout 2
30 min	30 min	30 min	30 min		30 min	30 min

▶ FOOD FOR THOUGHT
The real deal on protein and health.

Adding more protein to your diet makes good sense for weight control. In comparison with carbohydrate and fat, protein makes us feel more satisfied immediately after eating and reduces hunger between meals. In addition, protein increases our metabolic rate for one to three hours after eating. This means we burn more energy by the minute compared with the increase that occurs after eating carbs or fat. Protein foods are also excellent sources of micronutrients such as iron, zinc, vitamin B_{12}, and omega-3 fats.

Which foods are high in protein?
The best sources of protein are meats (beef, pork, lamb), chicken, fish, and shellfish. As long as these are trimmed of fat and not covered with creamy sauces, you can basically eat to suit your appetite. You will find there are natural limits on your appetite for lean protein. Go for the leanest cuts in the supermarket, cut off all the visible fat, and pan-fry, grill, bake, stir-fry, or barbecue.

Dairy products are not only good sources of protein, but the combination of protein and calcium that is unique to dairy foods can aid weight control. The more calcium or dairy foods (it's hard to separate the two) people eat, the lower their weight and fat mass. Calcium is intimately involved in the burning of fat—and that is something we want to encourage! Choose low-fat dairy products, including milk, yogurt, and cottage cheese. Though you don't have to cut them out completely, go easy on high-fat cheeses such as cheddar, feta, camembert, and brie. It is preferable to have a small serving of these than a giant serving of some reduced-fat version that doesn't taste anywhere near as good.

Nuts are excellent sources of protein and micronutrients, but we have to be careful not to overdo them, as they are energy dense—they pack a lot of calories into a small weight. While it is easy to overeat nuts, don't avoid them. They are high in the good fats. People who eat a small serving of nuts each day have significantly less risk of heart disease. We suggest you eat about 1 ounce most days. Put a small handful in a small bowl—don't eat straight from the pack.

It's a great shame that eggs have an undeserved bad reputation because of their cholesterol content—in fact they are great sources of protein and several essential vitamins and minerals. We now know that high blood cholesterol results from eating large amounts of saturated fat (rather than cholesterol) in foods. If you select the "omega-3-enriched" eggs on the market, you are boosting the good fats along with your protein intake.

Can you eat too much protein?

The American Institute of Medicine recommends that no more than 35 percent of energy in our diets come from protein. That is 175 grams of pure protein for a person consuming 2,000 calories a day. In practice, most people will have no desire to eat beyond that amount.

A high protein intake has been criticized because it might also mean a high intake of saturated fat. That won't be true if you stick to lean meat and low-fat dairy products. Concerns about the effects of high protein intake on kidney function are limited to people who already have compromised kidney function: people with diabetes, the very elderly, and infants.

	BREAKFAST	**SNACK**
MONDAY	Muesli with fruit and low-fat yogurt	Whole-grain cracker and peanut butter
TUESDAY	Whole-grain toast spread with avocado and topped with lean grilled bacon and sliced fresh tomato	An apple
WEDNESDAY	Commercial breakfast drink and a nut bar	Snack pack of peaches
THURSDAY	Whole-grain toast with peanut butter, pure honey, and sliced banana	Low-fat yogurt
FRIDAY	Fresh or canned fruit salad with low-fat natural yogurt and a sprinkle of mixed nuts and seeds	Raisin toast with a light spread of canola margarine
SATURDAY	Black bean omelet	A handful of dried apricots
SUNDAY	Grilled tomato, egg, and whole-grain toast	A banana

LUNCH	SNACK	DINNER
Toasted cheese and apple sandwich	Low-fat chocolate mousse	Tuna pasta with tomato and cucumber salad
Plain hamburger with lettuce, tomato, beets, onion, and sauce	Low-fat yogurt and fresh fruit	Chicken Stuffed with Spinach and Cheese (see page 249) served with sweet potato mash
Vegetable kebab with falafel and tabbouleh	Snack-size (25–30 grams) chocolate bar	Home-made fried rice using basmati rice
Whole-grain sandwich with ham and salad	A fresh pear	Spaghetti Bolognese: make your favorite Bolognese sauce with lean ground beef, allowing about 4 ounces of meat per person. Serve with spaghetti (1 cup cooked per person) and a big green side salad tossed in vinaigrette or balsamic dressing.
Chickpea salad: mix canned chickpeas, button mushrooms, diced red onion, pepper, parsley, and mint with vinaigrette dressing.	An apple	Pan-fry boneless fish fillets for 2–3 minutes on each side with a spray of olive oil. Serve with a squeeze of lemon, black pepper, and baby new potatoes, steamed broccoli florets, carrot, and asparagus spears.
Bruschetta with tomato topping and a frozen yogurt ice cream cone	An apple	Quick Thai noodle curry: stir-fry some diced trim tofu, sliced onion, red pepper strips, baby corn, and snow peas (or any stir-fry vegetable mix) in a large pan or wok. Add 1 tablespoon red curry paste. Prepare Asian noodles according to directions on the packet. Add the noodles to the vegetables with enough stock to make a sauce. Stir in 1 tablespoon light coconut milk, heat thoroughly, and serve.
Minestrone soup and a small whole-grain roll	Dried fruit and nut mix	Barbecued steak with corn, tomato, mushrooms, and salad

WEEK 6

This week is all about changing your thinking on fats and seeing the good as well as the bad. Focus on the following goals this week:

▶ **FOOD GOAL**

Break out of the "low-fat" dieting mentality.

▶ **EXERCISE GOAL**

Aim to walk at the same pace as last week (level 4 on the PRE scale) for a total of 20 minutes on six days. *Plus* try to complete each of the two resistance workouts, focusing on the upper and lower body respectively, three times during the week.

▶ **ACTIVITY GOAL**

For every hour that you spend sitting down, get up and do something more active for five minutes—have a quick stretch, walk to the printer, hang up the washing, or complete some other household or office chore.

▶ **FOOD FOR THOUGHT**

The fats of the matter.

▶ FOOD GOAL
Break out of the "low-fat" dieting mentality.

Your food goal this week involves looking at the fats in your diet—not to discard them, but to ensure that you are eating the right balance of good and bad fats. By allowing yourself to incorporate healthy fats into your diet, you will enjoy your meals more (fat tastes good) and gain the long-term benefits of fat-soluble vitamins and antioxidants. The following are the guidelines we recommend.

Eat less saturated fat
Reducing your total fat intake will lower the energy density of your diet and help you lose weight, but it is important to focus on specifically reducing the saturated fats as your highest priority. Saturated fats should constitute less than 10 percent of your total calories for the day. For a person eating 1,500 calories, this means eating less than 16 grams of saturated fat per day. (See table on page 112.)

Boost your omega-3 intake
These unique fats, found in seafood, can reduce inflammation in the body, iron out irregularities in heartbeat, and reduce blood-fat levels, and might play a valuable role in treating depression and Alzheimer's disease. Modern Western diets almost certainly do not provide enough of the polyunsaturated omega-3 fats. Around 650 milligrams of omega-3 fats is considered an adequate daily intake for adults. The following foods contain approximately 650 milligrams of omega-3 fats:

- 1½ ounces canned sardines
- 1 ounce canned mackerel
- 1½ ounces smoked salmon
- 1 ounce canned red salmon
- 1½ ounces canned pink salmon
- 4 ounces fresh Atlantic salmon
- 6 ounces canned tuna
- 4 omega-3 eggs

Replace bad fats with good fats
Replacing saturated fats with monounsaturated fats will lower your bad cholesterol and increase your good cholesterol.

▶ Substitute butter with canola margarines and spreads.

▶ Use liquid oils (or oil-based sprays) for frying, including canola and olive oils.

▶ Use cold-pressed olive oil, which contains antioxidants that are not found in refined oils.

▶ Check for the presence of healthy oils (canola or olive) in commercially fried and "oven-bake" products (if you use them), in preference to animal fats and unspecified vegetable oils.

▶ Use low-fat milk (or soy substitute) in place of whole milk.

▶ Eat a handful of nuts as an alternative to potato chips and other commercial bagged snacks.

Grams of saturated fat found in everyday servings of common foods

Chicken drumstick, 1 including skin	4 g
Cream cheese, 1 oz.	4 g
Sausage, 1 thin	4 g
Milk chocolate, 4 squares, 1 oz.	5 g
Pizza, supreme, 2 slices	5 g
Sour cream, 1 tablespoon	5 g
Cream, 1 tablespoon	6 g
Lamb loin chop (not trimmed), 1 grilled	6 g
Milk, full fat, 1 cup	6 g
Rich chocolate cake, iced and filled, 1 piece, 3½ oz.	6 g
Salami, 2 thin slices	6 g
Cheddar cheese, 1½ oz.	7 g
Chips, 1¾ oz. bag	7 g
Hamburger, 1 average	7 g
Shortbread, 3 biscuits	7 g
Butter, 1 tablespoon	10 g
Croissant, 1	10 g
Doughnut, 1 cinnamon and sugar	10 g
Meat pie, 1	10 g
Cheesecake, 1 large slice, 4¼ oz.	12 g
Sausage roll, 1 small	17 g
Fried chicken take-out meal, average	25 g

▶ EXERCISE GOAL

Aim to walk at the same pace as last week (level 4 on the PRE scale) for a total of 20 minutes on six days. *Plus* try to complete each of the two resistance workouts, focusing on the upper and lower body respectively, three times during the week.

Resistance exercises

This week, we make the resistance exercises you have already learned a little harder by omitting the rest between sets.

Workout 1	Lower-body exercises	"Core" strength abdominals and back
	Squats 1 set of 20	Three-quarter hover 2 x 30 seconds
	Lunges 10 each leg	Pointer 10 each side
Workout 2	Upper-body exercises	
	Assisted push-ups 1 set of 20	Leg extensions 10 each leg
	Standing tricep extensions 1 set of 20	Ab curl 1 set of 20

NEW EXERCISE

Ab curl

Now that we have started to strengthen the deep abdominal muscles involved in posture and support of the lower back, we can add an exercise for the outer muscles. A basic ab curl works the six-pack—the ab muscles that you use to sit up from lying down or to curl the torso forward. It is crucial to continue working the core muscles as well, so that you strengthen and tone from the inside out. The old-fashioned ab curl you may remember from school days (where you hooked your feet under a bar and sat up all the way) is not a good idea—this simply pulls your hip flexor muscles into play instead of making the abs do all the work.

Note: If you don't use great care, this exercise can strain the back and neck.

Strengthens and tones: the six-pack abs

How to do it:

1. Lie on the floor with your knees bent and your feet flat on the floor.
2. Lightly place your fingertips behind your ears and keep your elbows pointing to the side to avoid pulling on your head and neck.
3. Pull in your navel and curl your torso up about 45 degrees, then return to the floor.

Remember:

1. Keep the small of the back in contact with the floor.
2. Imagine you are holding an orange under your chin to maintain a space between your chin and chest.
3. Keep your eyes focused diagonally over your knees rather than looking straight up at the ceiling—a good place to look is where the ceiling meets the wall.

How many: 20 curls

Sample journal

Monday	Tuesday	Wednesday	Thursday	Friday	Saturday	Sunday
20 min walk	20 min walk	20 min walk	20 min walk		20 min walk	20 min walk
+ workout 1	+ workout 2	+ workout 1	+ workout 2		+ workout 1	+ workout 2
30 min	30 min	30 min	30 min		30 min	30 min

▶ FOOD FOR THOUGHT

The fats of the matter.

To most people, "low-fat" is still synonymous with "healthy" and "weight loss." Unfortunately, it is not that simple. Once upon a time, when fruit, vegetables, and whole grains were the staples of a low-fat diet, this might have been true. But it is no longer so—indeed, today's typical low-fat diet may be distinctly unhealthy—and one of the causes of our expanding waistlines.

In the 1990s, the experts told us to eat low-fat diets because they were concerned about two things. First, they believed saturated fat increased the risk of heart disease, and second, that fatty foods were too easily overeaten because they were energy dense. Those concerns are still valid today—the experts haven't changed their minds again. But the solution to the problem—eating a low-fat diet—has not been successful. While we have cut down on total fat, we haven't cut down on saturated fat, and the food industry (with the best of intentions) gave us a myriad of low-fat foods that were just as energy dense as their full-fat counterparts. So, during the 1990s, the era of "99 percent fat-free," the prevalence of obesity soared and with it, heart disease and diabetes.

As a result of these unexpected events, the heart foundations and health organizations around the world went back to the drawing board and remodeled their dietary advice, as follows:

1. The *type* of fat is more important for health than the total amount.
2. The energy density of a food (calories per 100 grams) is more important to weight control than the fat content.

Furthermore, most of us need to eat more of certain kinds of fat for optimal health (yes, you read it right). These include the omega-3 fats found in fish and seafood, walnuts, and canola-based products. Eating these along with more monounsaturated fats, such as those in olive oil and canola oil, has been shown to reduce the risk of heart attack significantly. Indeed, one of the most important diet studies ever carried out, the Lyon Heart Study, showed that a diet with more fish, fruit, vegetables, and good fats was twice as effective in reducing cardiovascular "events" as the low-fat diet recommended by the American Heart Association. In fact, it is a whole lot better than most of the expensive drugs used to reduce the risk of heart attack.

There is another excellent reason why you should aim to increase these monounsaturated fats at the expense of the saturated ones. While all fats have the same number of calories per gram, they may not all have the same effect on your weight. For reasons that are not yet clear, a high-fat diet based on fish oil or olive oil is much less likely to expand the waistline. Research also shows that people who eat diets rich in the omega-3 fats are less likely to suffer rheumatoid arthritis, psoriasis, ulcerative colitis, depression (and other mental illness), and possibly some cancers. We recommend that you eat the food fats in the form of food rather than pills or just oils. In the whole food, you get the whole package that nature provided.

Where do you find the good oils?
- Fish such as salmon, tuna, herrings, and sardines—canned or fresh
- Shellfish
- Walnuts, almonds, and cashews—best unsalted
- Avocado—spread it on as an alternative to margarine or butter
- Spinach, bok choy, leafy green salads
- Olives—spread as a tapenade or add whole to almost anything —pasta sauces, couscous, or salads
- Muesli—mix sunflower seeds and pumpkin seeds with ground almonds or hazelnuts
- Linseed (flaxseed) is a great source of omega-3 fats; a good way to eat it is in soy-and-linseed bread

■

A LOW-FAT DIET
IS NOT NECESSARILY THE BEST DIET
FOR WEIGHT LOSS OR OVERALL HEALTH.

"FAT-FREE" AND "REDUCED-FAT"
ON THE LABEL IS NOT A
LICENSE TO EAT MORE.

EATING LESS SATURATED FAT
AND MORE MONOUNSATURATED
AND OMEGA-3 FATS
IS THE BEST OPTION
FOR LONG-TERM HEALTH.

■

WEEK 6 MENU PLAN

	BREAKFAST	SNACK
MONDAY	Orange and grapefruit segments with prunes and a low-fat honey-flavored yogurt, sprinkled with toasted flaked almonds	Raisin toast
TUESDAY	Soy-and-linseed toast with margarine and a boiled egg, plus a cup of coffee with low-fat milk	A banana
WEDNESDAY	Muesli with sliced pear and low-fat milk, sprinkled with chopped almonds or hazelnuts	A small vegetable juice, whole-grain crackers
THURSDAY	Banana smoothie made with an omega-3 egg	Hot chocolate with low-fat milk
FRIDAY	Toasted cheese and tomato sandwich and an apple	Low-fat yogurt
SATURDAY	High-fiber, low-GI cereal with low-fat milk and canned peach slices	Dried fruit cookies
SUNDAY	Egg, lean bacon, tomato, mushrooms, and whole-grain toast with grapefruit juice	An apple

LUNCH	SNACK	DINNER
Miso soup with sushi rolls	An apple	Stir-fried beef with garlic, onion, pepper, carrot, zucchini, and snow peas dressed with sweet chili sauce and served with basmati rice
Chicken and coleslaw on a mixed-grain roll with fresh or canned fruit salad	Low-fat chocolate milk	Spread a round of pita bread with pesto or tomato paste. Top with sliced tomato, mushrooms, roasted pepper, black olives, chopped spring onions, and a sprinkle of grated Parmesan cheese. Heat up in a hot oven.
Salmon and lettuce sandwich on whole-grain bread	2 kiwi fruit	Beef stroganoff with mushrooms (substitute light sour cream for sour cream) with fettuccine, steamed broccoli, and cauliflower
Lean ham, pineapple, and grated light cheese on a toasted mixed-grain muffin	An orange	Commercial oven-bake fish and potato wedges with carrot and zucchini julienne
Steak sandwich made on whole-grain bread with salad	A banana	Thai-style Tofu and Noodle Soup (see page 252)
Minestrone soup and a crusty white roll	An apple	Thinly slice and pan-fry pork loin steak. Toss with baby spinach, sliced red onion, and steamed new potatoes (halved or quartered).
Macaroni and cheese made with light milk and reduced-fat cheese. Throw in a bag of frozen mixed vegetables with the macaroni.	Snack-size chocolate bar (1 ounce)	Roast leg of lamb with a small roast potato, roast sweet potato, pumpkin, string beans, and peas, served with mint sauce

WEEK 7

This week, focus on these goals:

▶ FOOD GOAL
Think about what you are drinking.

▶ EXERCISE GOAL
Aim to walk at the same pace as last week (level 4 on the PRE scale), but for a total of 25 minutes on six days. *Plus* try to complete each of the two resistance workouts, focusing on the upper and lower body respectively, three times during the week.

▶ ACTIVITY GOAL
Watch no more than two hours of television on any day and choose one day when you will not watch television at all.

▶ FOOD FOR THOUGHT
Whole grains—the whole story.

▶ FOOD GOAL
Think about what you are drinking.

Did you know that it's a good idea to drink more when you are losing weight? One reason is that a large part of our fluid intake comes from food, so if we are eating less food, we are also taking in less fluid. Additional fluid is also helpful for removing extra toxins that can be released during weight loss. What you choose to drink, however, can have a major impact on your success with weight loss.

Many things we drink would be better thought of as food due to the amount of calories they contain. Fruit juice might sound like a healthy option, but ordering a glass of orange juice in a café can be the equivalent of the energy (calories) from ten oranges; a large soft drink can provide as many as 15 teaspoons of sugar in a single serving; and a take-out coffee can contain as much as 10 grams of fat if made with whole milk. It is not hard to see how the calories can stack up without filling you up.

Of all the things we drink, however, alcohol could be thought of as the most fattening—not because of its calorie content, but because it has priority as a fuel over all other nutrients. This means that as long as there is alcohol in your system, anything else is surplus until the alcohol calories are used up. Looking at it another way, just one can of beer replaces all the calories burned by twenty minutes of brisk walking.

Your best option for extra fluid is water. Soda water, low-sodium mineral water, herbal teas, and decaffeinated drinks are other good options. Diet soft drinks are okay—certainly they contain almost no calories, but they are highly acidic (which can soften the enamel of your teeth). Plus, be aware of the caffeine content in these types of drinks, which can be considerable.

When you are trying to lose weight, it is best to think of alcohol as an indulgence. It may be enjoyable, but it doesn't provide any essential nutrients and is high in calories. Limit your intake as much as you can. Even when you get to the weight-maintenance stage, an average daily limit of no more than two standard drinks for men and one standard drink for women is recommended.

A standard drink is:

▶ 4 ounces of wine
▶ 10 ounces of wine cooler

▶ 12 ounces of beer
▶ 1¼ ounces of distilled liquor
▶ 2 ounces of fortified wine (sherry, port, etc.)

Did you know?

Your body reacts differently to fluids than it does to food. There is evidence that sugar in liquid form (such as soft drinks and fruit juices) may sneak past the brain's appetite center. When we chew, signals are sent to the brain that food is on its way and our appetite begins to be altered before the food even hits our stomach. When we drink, however, these signals don't occur, and the same level of satiety is not reached, making it easy for us to consume too much.

▶ EXERCISE GOAL

Aim to walk at the same pace as last week (level 4 on the PRE scale), but for a total of 25 minutes on six days. *Plus* try to complete each of the two resistance workouts, focusing on the upper and lower body respectively, three times during the week.

Resistance exercises

Workout 1	Lower-body exercises	"Core" strength abdominals and back
	Squats 1 set of 20	Three-quarter hover 2 x 30 seconds
	Lunges 10 each leg	Pointer 10 each side
Workout 2	**Upper-body exercises**	
	Assisted push-ups 1 set of 20	Leg extensions 10 each leg
	Standing tricep extensions 1 set of 20	Ab curl 1 set of 20
	Bicep curl 1 set of 20	

NEW EXERCISE

Bicep curl

When working one muscle or group of muscles, we should always try to work the opposing muscle(s) to the same extent. This maintains an equilibrium of strength and flexibility across joints and is crucial to achieving good posture and avoiding injuries. We learned to work the back of the arm last week; therefore, this week we need to add an exercise for the front of the arm. A bicep curl is the most effective and simple way to do this.

Strengthens and tones: the front of the arm

How to do it:
1. Hold your hand weights (or cans) by your sides with your palms facing forward.
2. Maintain good posture through your body, keeping your torso strong and upright throughout.
3. Curl the weights up toward your shoulders, keeping your elbows close to your rib cage, and slowly return to the start position.

How many: Complete 20 curls

Sample journal

Monday	Tuesday	Wednesday	Thursday	Friday	Saturday	Sunday
25 min walk	25 min walk	25 min walk	25 min walk		25 min walk	25 min walk
+ workout 1	+ workout 2	+ workout 1	+ workout 2		+ workout 1	+ workout 2
35 min	35 min	35 min	35 min		35 min	35 min

■

A BICEP CURL IS THE MOST EFFECTIVE AND SIMPLE WAY TO STRENGTHEN AND TONE THIS PART OF THE ARM.

■

▶ FOOD FOR THOUGHT
Whole grains—the whole story.

While there is plenty of evidence that whole grains and cereal fiber are good for you, there are plenty of nutritious foods that are relatively low in fiber and yet full of micronutrients (such as oranges, dairy products, fish, and lean meat). In our experience, only a small minority of people are willing to eat cereal products in their true "native state." For many people, unrefined foods, such as brown bread, brown rice, and brown pasta, are not to their liking.

Humans did not eat large amounts of any cereal grain until the advent of agriculture, a recent event on the evolutionary time line. But once farming became established, we found increasingly ingenious ways of removing the "brown bits" and making cereal products ever more palatable—probably too palatable for our own good!

Having said this, the benefits of eating more fiber—especially if you are battling the bulge—are obvious. In one study of nearly 3,000 young adults, those who ate more fiber (about 25 grams a day) gained much less weight over the years than those who ate the least (less than 10 grams a day). What's more, their fiber intake was a better predictor of the amount of weight gain than their fat intake (the usual suspect). Why? Lots of reasons: high-fiber foods take longer to eat, they are heavier and bulkier, fill you up sooner, and leave you feeling more satiated (think of grainy bread versus white bread). Another reason is that eating more whole grains and fiber has been shown to improve insulin sensitivity and lower insulin levels. That means greater use of fat as a source of fuel—good news if you are trying to lose weight.

There are plenty of other reasons to encourage you to eat more whole grains if you enjoy them. Higher fiber intake—especially from cereals—has been linked to lower risk of cancer of the large bowel, breast, stomach, and mouth. What is the connection? New research shows that high insulin levels increase the multiplication of mutated cells, producing uncontrolled growth of tumors and cancers. Plus, another function of fiber is to bind carcinogenic substances and help sweep them out of the system.

Much of the goodness in grains is found just beneath the bran layer and is usually lost along with the fiber when grains are milled. Vitamins, minerals, antioxidants, and other protective substances in whole grains—many of which are not present in nutritional supplements—are also lost. However, some wheats are better than others—when hard wheats, such as durum wheat, are milled into flour or semolina (to make pasta), it is easier to separate the bran, and the final product contains higher quantities of micronutrients.

Our take-home message is to reduce your intake of highly processed and refined cereal products that produce glycemic spikes and leave you craving more. The most obvious examples are soft white bread and low-fat snacks and crackers, but there are also some foods that are high in fiber—modern whole-meal breads (where you can't see the grain) and brown rice, for example, that are quickly digested and absorbed. We recommend you swap some of these high-GI carbohydrates for smart carbs that are slowly digested and absorbed, regardless of their fiber content. Pasta, noodles, low-GI rice varieties, and sourdough bread are good examples of low-GI foods that everyone enjoys. While their fiber content may be low, some of the starch is resistant to digestion and aids large-bowel health in the same way that fiber does. If you enjoy the high-fiber version, that's an added bonus!

If a food's label shows at least 3 grams of fiber per serving, consider it a good source. Experts recommend 30 grams of fiber a day. Increase your fiber intake slowly so your bowel flora has time to adapt.

Low-GI sources of fiber (grams per serving)

Grain bread (lots of whole kernels visible), 1 slice	2 g
Old-fashioned oatmeal, 1 cup, cooked	2 g
Apple, 1 medium, including skin	3 g
Barley, ½ cup, cooked	3 g
Corn, 3½ ounces, canned	3 g
Lentils, ½ cup, cooked	3 g
Prunes, 5	3 g
Sweet potato, 4 ounces, boiled	3 g
Popcorn, 2 cups, popped	4 g
Pumpernickel bread, 1¾ slice	4 g
Dried apricots, 6 halves	5 g
Peas, ½ cup, cooked	5 g
All-Bran, ½ cup	10 g
Chickpeas, ½ cup, cooked	10 g

WEEK 7 MENU PLAN

	BREAKFAST	SNACK
MONDAY	Whole-grain bread spread with fresh ricotta and blackberry preserve	A banana
TUESDAY	Breakfast on the Go (see page 230)	Skim-milk latte
WEDNESDAY	Low-GI, high-fiber breakfast cereal with low-fat milk and sliced banana	Mandarins
THURSDAY	Low-fat toasted muesli with yogurt and canned fruit	An apple
FRIDAY	Fruit bread spread with light cream cheese and topped with sliced apple and a sprinkle of cinnamon	Dried pear halves
SATURDAY	Mushroom, cheese, and spinach omelet with whole-grain toast and a glass of fruit juice	An apple
SUNDAY	Chopped banana stirred into oatmeal, topped with a drizzle of honey and low-fat milk	Oatmeal cookies

LUNCH	SNACK	DINNER
Pasta salad with lean ham, corn kernels, pepper, shallots, and mayonnaise with lettuce	Low-fat yogurt	Stir-fry lean beef with grated ginger and crushed garlic. Add snow peas, broccoli florets, chopped spring onion, Chinese cabbage slices, and a little finely chopped chili. Combine soy and hoisin sauces with honey, toss and serve with basmati rice.
Asian seafood combination with vegetables and boiled noodles	Canned peaches	Pan-fried chicken breast with mushroom sauce (use light evaporated milk in place of cream), canned butter beans, carrots, and green beans
Chicken, avocado, and salad on whole-grain bread	Low-fat fruit yogurt	Boil a package of spinach and cheese (or your favorite filling) tortellini according to package directions. Heat some bottled tomato sauce and serve this on top of the tortellini with a sprinkle of Parmesan cheese. Serve with a large salad and vinaigrette dressing.
Whole-grain crackers with hummus, sliced tomato, celery, and sardines	Carrot sticks with hummus	Mediterranean roast vegetables with trimmed lamb cutlets
Pumpkin soup with whole-grain toasted croutons and low-fat yogurt garnish	Orange and Passion Fruit Mousse (see page 265)	Mexican bean tacos: fill warm taco shells with 2–3 tablespoons refried beans and top with shredded lettuce, grated reduced-fat cheese, and 1–2 teaspoons light sour cream.
Steak sandwich: grilled minute steak in multigrain bread with lettuce, beets, grated carrot, tomato, and mustard	A banana	Roasted rosemary sweet potato wedges with oven-baked fish. Brush sweet potato wedges with a little olive oil, sprinkle with dried rosemary, and bake in the oven for about 20 minutes at 350°F. Wrap fish fillets or cutlets (allowing one per person) in individual foil parcels with a slice or two of lemon and a twist of freshly ground black pepper, and bake in the oven for 10 to 15 minutes.
Sardines or smoked trout, sourdough bread, and fresh green salad with lemon and vinegar	Baked banana with passion fruit (try it in the microwave)	Ham and Vegetable Bake (see page 236) and salad

WEEK 8

Many of us assign foods to a "good" or "bad" category, and inevitably it is the foods we see as treat foods that we see as "bad." Yet by allowing yourself to indulge in whatever food and drink you really enjoy, you can diminish the uncontrollable desire to overeat these foods, and they become a normal part of eating. Focus on the following goals this week:

▶ FOOD GOAL
Include an indulgence occasionally.

▶ EXERCISE GOAL
Aim to walk for a total of 25 minutes on six days, but increase your pace to a brisk walk (of around level 5 on the PRE scale) for the middle 15 minutes. *Plus* try to complete each of the resistance workouts, focusing on the upper and lower body respectively, three times during the week.

▶ ACTIVITY GOAL
Go shopping on foot and carry your bags home—a fantastic total body workout! (If you have to drive to the nearest shopping center, park the car in the farthest parking spot and walk the rest of the way.)

▶ FOOD FOR THOUGHT
Allow yourself something sweet!

▶ FOOD GOAL

Include an indulgence occasionally.

Do you usually finish your main course and find yourself hankering for a little something sweet? Do you prefer your tea and coffee with the taste of real sugar? Perhaps you feel that a sweet fix helps you work through the afternoon. Maybe you really enjoy coffee and cake with a good friend once a week. Bad habits? We don't think so.

Just because you have decided to change your eating habits doesn't mean you can't indulge once a week. Imagine that you are at a meeting and suddenly a chocolate mud cake is being offered around. It is okay to enjoy a piece of cake with everyone else, but make the decision to eat—or not eat—an active one. Do you automatically accept a piece of cake (even though you're not hungry) and eat it during the meeting, barely tasting it (passively indulging)? Or do you consider the look of the cake and how hungry you are and decide it could be a nice change for a morning snack (actively making a decision)? Your thoughts and actions in the second instance are more positive than in the first instance, which means you are less likely to feel guilty about indulging.

Indulgences to savor:

3 fruit-filled cookies

½ slice of cake

2 cream-filled cookies

1 ounce of your favorite cheese

1 snack-size (1 ounce) chocolate bar

2 glasses (8 ounces) wine

2 tablespoons cream

½ small serving french fries

12-ounce beer

In the era of digital cameras, it's easy to take a weekly snapshot of your body (full length) in profile. Take it in the same place each week (such as inside a door frame) so you can easily see your weekly progress.

This week, we want you to look at the feelings you may have about eating certain foods. The aim is for you to make active, guilt-free choices about the foods you eat, confident in the knowledge that you can eat your favorite foods and still work toward your goals. This is also a good time to revise your basic daily food quantities to be sure your background diet is sound. (See pages 60–61.)

And in case you haven't done so for a while, this week, choose an indulgence that you crave and go ahead and enjoy it!

▶ EXERCISE GOAL

Aim to walk for a total of 25 minutes on six days, but increase your pace to a brisk walk (of around level 5 on the PRE scale) for the middle 15 minutes. *Plus* try to complete each of the resistance workouts, focusing on the upper and lower body respectively, three times during the week.

Resistance exercises

Workout 1	Lower-body exercises	"Core" strength abdominals and back
	Squats 1 set of 20	Full hover 2 x 30 seconds
	Lunges 10 each leg	Pointer 10 each side
	Power lunge 20 alternate legs	
Workout 2	**Upper-body exercises**	
	Assisted push-ups 1 set of 20	Leg extensions 10 each leg
	Standing tricep extensions 1 set of 20	Ab curl 1 set of 20
	Bicep curl 1 set of 20	

NEW EXERCISES

Power lunges

This is a more advanced version of the lunge you have already learned. By adding some movement, you recruit all the smaller stabilizer muscles of the legs, the postural muscles have to work hard, and you increase the load the major muscles of the legs and bottom have to move. This is a fantastic exercise for toning and strengthening the lower body.

Strengthens and tones: legs and bottom

How to do it:
1. Start with your feet hip-width apart and your arms by your side. Keep your eyes looking straight ahead rather than down at the floor to help you maintain good posture.
2. Take a long step forward with one leg and sink into your usual lunge, but then push yourself back to standing by driving into your front heel.
3. As you complete the power lunge, allow your arms to swing naturally by your sides to help with balance. Repeat on the other leg.

Remember: Keep your chest proud and upper body upright throughout so that all the work is done by the legs and bottom muscles.
How many: 20, using alternate legs

Full hover
This is a more advanced level of the three-quarter hover you have already learned.

Strengthens and tones: core abdominals—improves your posture and narrows your waist

How to do it:
1. Start in your three-quarter hover position (see page 96) and then lift your knees, straightening your legs until your body is in alignment from heel to shoulder.
2. Check that your bottom is not sticking up and that you are not allowing your lower back to sag—pull your navel in toward your spine.
3. Straighten up and keep your hips in line with your body.

Remember: Breathe normally while you maintain the position—it is very easy to hold your breath without realizing it.
How long: Hold for 2 sets of 30 seconds with a short rest in between.

Sample journal

Monday	Tuesday	Wednesday	Thursday	Friday	Saturday	Sunday
25 min walk	25 min walk	25 min walk	25 min walk		25 min walk	25 min walk
+ workout 1	+ workout 2	+ workout 1	+ workout 2		+ workout 1	+ workout 2
35 min	35 min	35 min	35 min		35 min	35 min

▶ FOOD FOR THOUGHT
Allow yourself something sweet!

Most people mistakenly believe that sugar is the first thing that ought to go when they are "on a diet"—it is just "empty calories" and is probably responsible for one's current state of overweight. We tend to have a prudish notion that if something tastes good, it must be bad for us. However, yearning for something sweet is instinctual and hard to ignore, especially when you are actively losing weight. In our evolutionary past, honey was a significant part of hunter-gatherer diets and a lot more concentrated as a source of sugar than most of the sugary foods we eat today.

In fact, sugar is not specifically implicated in making us fat. In the Baltimore Aging Study, for example, the best predictor of weight gain over time was a diet characterized by a lot of bread (most varieties of which were high-GI). Those who ate a lot of sweets gained very little— about the same as those who adhered to the principles of healthy eating (lots of fruit, vegetables, whole grains, and lean protein).

It is obvious, too, that the vast array of sugar-free and "no added sugar" foods on supermarket shelves has not solved the problem of overweight. In fact, it could be said that they have exacerbated the problem by encouraging people to think that using a sugar substitute is all it takes to cut calories and control weight. If only!

Here is a word of caution, however. If, for example, you give people 500 extra calories as solid food, they compensate by consuming fewer calories during the rest of the day. But if you feed them 500 calories in a soft drink, juice, or other clear liquid, they don't reduce their intake at all. All 500 calories are surplus, and may head straight for your hips or waist. Indeed, in a recent study, the children who became overweight were greater consumers of soft drinks and fruit juices than the children who did not.

In the Low GI Diet Revolution, we encourage you to enjoy refined sugar in moderation—that's about 40 to 50 grams a day, an amount that most people consume without even thinking about it. Include sweetened foods that contain nutrients, not just calories—dairy foods, breakfast cereals, hot cereal with brown sugar, or jam on whole-grain toast. Even the World Health Organization says, "A moderate intake of sugar-rich foods can provide for a palatable and nutritious diet." We want you to cut the guilt trip and allow yourself the pleasure of sweetness. To guide you, let's take a quick look at the sugar content of some common foods.

Refined sugar content of various foods

1 shortbread cookie	3 g
1 cream-filled cookie	5 g
1 cup sweetened fruit juice	5 g
1 rounded teaspoon sugar	6 g
1 cinnamon and sugar doughnut	7 g
1 piece unfrosted vanilla cake	7 g
1 tablespoon jam	8 g
1 muesli bar (average)	8 g
1 piece chocolate cake	11 g
1 ounce undiluted cordial	18 g
5 squares chocolate	20 g
1 tablespoon honey	20 g
1 chocolate bar (average)	35 g
12-ounce can soft drink (average)	45 g

WEEK 8 MENU PLAN

	BREAKFAST	SNACK
MONDAY	High-fiber fruit smoothie: blend low-fat milk, natural yogurt, a banana, a handful of berries, and 1 tablespoon psyllium husks.	A small handful of raw almonds
TUESDAY	1 cup bean soup with 3 whole-grain crackers	An apple and a wedge of reduced-fat cheddar
WEDNESDAY	Grilled lean bacon and tomato sandwich on sourdough bread	A handful of red grapes
THURSDAY	Traditional oatmeal served with low-fat milk and a dollop of raspberry jam	Hot chocolate with low-fat milk
FRIDAY	Home-made muesli (blend of rolled oats, mixture of dried fruit, nuts, and seeds) with low-fat milk and a few sliced strawberries	Low-fat fruit yogurt
SATURDAY	Egg and bacon with toast, tomato, and mushroom	An apple
SUNDAY	Omelet filled with spinach and mushrooms served with toasted sourdough bread	Skim-milk latte with a small piece of unfrosted vanilla cake

LUNCH	SNACK	DINNER
Lean ham and lots of salad veggies—lettuce, tomato, beets, grated carrot, and sprouts—on whole-grain bread, flavored with mustard or chutney	A piece of fruit	Spaghetti Bolognese made with lean beef—serve with a large mixed salad, a shaving of Parmesan, and a small glass of red wine
Tortilla wrap filled with chicken, lettuce, tomato, cucumber, and salsa	A small (1-ounce) chocolate bar	Herbed Fish Parcels with Sweet Potato Wedges and Coleslaw (see page 253)
Tomato and barley soup with whole-grain bread and low-fat cheese	Skim-milk hot chocolate	Chicken and cashew nut stir-fry with pepper, mushrooms, onion, ginger, garlic, chili, Asian greens, and 1 teaspoon honey, served with noodles or basmati rice
Smoked mackerel fillet with a large mixed salad and a slice of sourdough bread, plus a piece of fresh fruit	Your favorite ice cream	Grilled lean beef steak with a steamed ear of corn and a large mixed salad dressed with a little olive oil and vinegar dressing
Roast beef sandwich on whole-grain bread with salad vegetables and mustard	Peaches and cream	Salad Niçoise with lettuce, blanched green beans, boiled new potatoes, hard-boiled egg, olives, spring onions, baby gherkins, anchovies, and plum tomatoes. Top with fresh or canned tuna and drizzle with olive oil and lemon juice dressing.
Mixed-bean salad with watercress and a slice of whole-grain bread	A handful of red grapes	Seafood fettuccine in a tomato-based sauce and a green salad
Barbecued Lamb with Lentil Salad and Lemon-Yogurt Dressing (see page 250)	Fruit salad with natural yogurt	Quick pita bread pizza: top a pita bread with tomato paste, chopped zucchini, pepper, tomato, and mixed herbs, sprinkle with reduced-fat mozzarella, and bake for 20 minutes in a hot oven. Serve with a green salad.

WEEK 9

After two months of changing your eating and exercise habits step by step, you should be feeling and looking lighter and brighter! If, however, you are finding your energy levels are lagging, it could be that you have cut your food intake too much—particularly your intake of carbohydrates. With this in mind, you should focus on the following goals this week:

▶ FOOD GOAL

Ensure you are eating enough carbohydrate (from low-GI sources) to give you the energy to sustain your increased exercise and activity levels.

▶ EXERCISE GOAL

Aim to walk for a total of 30 minutes on six days at the same brisk pace as last week (around level 5 on the PRE scale) for the middle 15 minutes. *Plus* try to complete each of the resistance workouts, focusing on the upper and lower body respectively, three times during the week.

▶ ACTIVITY GOAL

Instead of heading to the local car wash, do it yourself by hand, including an internal spring cleaning.

▶ FOOD FOR THOUGHT

Facts and fallacies about the GI.

▶ FOOD GOAL

Ensure you are eating enough carbohydrate (from low-GI sources) to give you the energy to sustain your increased exercise and activity levels.

While cutting out carbs might bring rapid results when you weigh yourself, such weight loss is inevitably too difficult to maintain long term. You need a certain amount of carbs to function at your best, particularly given your recent increased exercise and activity levels.

Focus this week on the carb-rich foods you are eating and assess whether you are including a low-GI carb in each meal. Your goal is not to load your body with a huge amount of carbohydrate in one meal, but to spread a moderate amount of slowly absorbed low-GI carbs to fuel your body across the course of the day. This translates into gentle fluctuations in your blood glucose, with less insulin being required to deal with the day's intake. Perhaps keep a journal for a few days and then look back to check on how you are really doing. If you find you are not spreading your carb intake across the day, try following our suggested meal plans for a few days.

Sample day (low-GI choices in italics to show servings spread throughout the day)

Breakfast: *natural muesli* with *low-fat milk* and sliced *fresh berries*
Snack: *banana* and a *low-fat yogurt*
Lunch: *lentil* soup with *low-GI bread* and reduced-fat cheese
Snack: hot chocolate made with *low-fat milk* and an *oatmeal cookie*
Dinner: grilled salmon fillet with baked *sweet potato* and a green salad

▶ EXERCISE GOAL

Aim to walk for a total of 30 minutes on six days at the same brisk pace as last week (around level 5 on the PRE scale) for the middle 15 minutes. *Plus* try to complete each of the resistance workouts, focusing on the upper and lower body respectively, three times during the week.

Most health authorities around the world agree that for health, we should aim to achieve 30 minutes of walking on most days of the week. This week our goal is to meet those recommendations. You are now well on your way to better health, a leaner body, and a more active mind—well done!

Resistance exercises

Workout 1	Lower-body exercises	"Core" strength abdominals and back
	Squats 1 set of 20	Full hover 2 x 30 seconds
	Lunges 10 each leg	Pointer 10 each side
	Power lunges 20 alternate legs	
Workout 2	**Upper-body exercises**	
	Three-quarter push-ups 1 set of 20	Leg extensions 10 each leg
	Standing tricep extensions 1 set of 20	Ab curl 1 set of 20
	Bicep curl 1 set of 20	Oblique curl 20 each side

NEW EXERCISES

Three-quarter push-ups

This uses the same technique as the assisted push-ups (pages 80–81), but we make things a little more challenging by removing the help of the table (or stair). Ensure you set up with a wide hand stance and keep your bottom tucked while you lower your chest to the floor.

Oblique curl

This is a variation of the ab curl that you have already learned (pages 113–14).

Strengthens and tones: waist and torso

How to do it:
1. From your ab curl position drop both knees down to the right.
2. Extend your left arm behind your body toward your left heel and reach for the heel as you curl the body up. Make sure you keep your shoulders square to the ceiling (you will feel like twisting in the direction of your knees) and use your right hand to lightly support the weight of your head to avoid straining your neck.

3. Repeat on the other side.

How Many: 20 curls on each side

Sample journal

Monday	Tuesday	Wednesday	Thursday	Friday	Saturday	Sunday
30 min walk	30 min walk	30 min walk	30 min walk		30 min walk	30 min walk
+ workout 2	+ workout 1	+ workout 2	+ workout 1		+ workout 2	+ workout 1
40 min	40 min	40 min	40 min		40 min	40 min

▶ FOOD FOR THOUGHT
Facts and fallacies about the GI.

1. **Carrots have a high GI value.**
No, they don't! They have a GI value of 41 and you can eat them as a "free food." The reason for the confusion: the first research ever published gave them a high GI (92). Unfortunately, it was based on too few subjects, and the resulting average was skewed. This error made the GI concept highly controversial right from the beginning.

2. **The GI doesn't consider the amount of carbohydrate in a serving of food.**
That's true—it is a measure of the carbohydrate quality, not quantity. Do we need to know the quantity, too? For the most part, no. If you substitute a low-GI bread for others, a low-GI breakfast cereal for others, and a low-GI rice for others, then you are achieving your goal: a low-GI diet in which the carbs are slowly digested and absorbed. If you are choosing chocolate over watermelon (not a good idea, really) then it is sensible to consider both quality and quantity (the glycemic load). For more on the glycemic load, see page 32.

3. **Some foods have a high GI but contain little carbohydrate.**
True. There are a handful of foods that contain so little carbohydrate that their GI value is irrelevant. These include watermelon and cantaloupe, pumpkin, parsnips, and fava beans. You can ignore their high GI.

4. **Glycemic load (GL) makes more sense than GI.**
Not true. The GI can be more important than the GL. That's

because it is critical to choose slowly digested carbs (low-GI carbs) over quickly digested ones (high-GI carbs), even if the GL is the same. You'll stay fuller longer if you choose a normal portion of pasta (a low-GI food) over a small serving of potato (a high-GI food). Our primary goal should be improving the quality of the carbs (exchanging high GI for low GI), not reducing the quantity of carbohydrate eaten. A secondary goal—it's up to you—is to replace some of the high-GI carbs with good fats or lean protein.

5. **Cutting carbs is the best way to lower insulin levels.**

No, that's not correct. While it is true that high-GI carbs produce high insulin responses, low-GI carbs have the same insulin demand as high-protein foods that contain no carbs. See the diagram on page 20. Moreover, people who eat more carbs have better insulin sensitivity than those who eat fewer carbs.

6. **Whole-wheat products have low GI values.**

Not true most of the time. Cereal products, especially those derived from wheat, usually have the same GI value as their white counterparts. For example, white bread's GI is 70; whole-wheat bread's GI is 71. One rule to follow is that if you can't see the whole or cracked grains, it's probably not low-GI, whatever it says on the package. When wheat bran is finely milled, digestive enzymes can attack fast. That's not to say whole-wheat cereals are unhealthy. There is good evidence that whole-wheat foods improve insulin sensitivity and reduce disease risk. The best choices are both low-GI and high in fiber.

7. **The GI doesn't work in mixed meals.**

Yes, it does—it works perfectly. Why the controversy? Early studies on the subject of mixed meals were carried out by vocal opponents of the GI concept. Subsequent studies—at least a dozen from all over the world—proved convincingly that the GI value of single foods could be used to predict the GI value of a mixed meal. Moreover, long-term studies comparing high- and low-GI diets show differences in measures of blood-glucose control. If the GI values of single foods were not a good guide to food choices, then those differences would not be evident.

8. **The GI doesn't work when you add protein or fat.**

Not true. When you add protein or fat to a high-carbohydrate food—for example, cheese to bread—the blood-glucose response will go down. But if you then exchange the source of carbohydrate (instead of bread with cheese, for example, you have pasta with cheese), then you can expect an even lower response. The relative ranking of carbohydrate foods according to their GI predicts the overall glycemic response even in the presence of extra protein and fat. There will be limits to this, of course—if your meal contains a lot of protein and fat and little in the way of carbs, then the GI becomes irrelevant.

9. **Too many variables affect the blood-glucose response to meals.**
It's true that many variables affect your glycemic response to meals. But that criticism applies as well to carbohydrate "counting" as it does to the GI. And carbohydrate counting is highly recommended for people with diabetes. Your day-to-day variation will be influenced by many things, including things you did the day before: amount of exercise; consumption of fat, fiber, and alcohol; and even amount of sleep. What's good to know is that a low-GI meal at dinner or breakfast will improve your glycemic response to lunch the following day, regardless of what you eat.

10. **Choosing low-GI foods takes precedence over any other consideration.**
Of course not! If you're under the illusion that chocolate's low GI value is a reason to go to town on it, think again. In recommending the GI, we don't want people to throw common sense to the wind. The GI is not meant to be used in isolation. Reducing saturated and trans fats is vitally important. Eat lots of fruit and veggies (except potatoes) for their vitamins, minerals, antioxidants, and fiber, and disregard their GI value. Cutting down on the volume of soft drinks, ice cream, cakes, cookies, and candy, regardless of their GI value, is important. That does not mean strict avoidance—remember, an indulgence a day keeps bingeing at bay. (That's especially true if your indulgence is low-GI to boot.)

WEEK 9 MENU PLAN

	BREAKFAST	SNACK
MONDAY	Natural muesli topped with sliced banana and natural yogurt	Low-fat drinkable yogurt
TUESDAY	Whole-grain toast with a skim of peanut butter	Low-fat flavored milk
WEDNESDAY	A low-GI cereal with low-fat milk and sliced strawberries	A pear
THURSDAY	Alpen muesli with sliced peach	A quarter of a honeydew melon
FRIDAY	Natural muesli with 1 tablespoon of blueberries and natural yogurt	A small handful of almonds
SATURDAY	Banana and Ricotta Toast (see page 261)	A handful of pistachio nuts in their shells
SUNDAY	Scrambled eggs with whole-grain toast, grilled tomato, and dry-fried mushrooms	A quarter of a cantaloupe

LUNCH	SNACK	DINNER
Sushi rolls and a bowl of miso soup	Apple slices and a chunk of reduced-fat cheddar	Lentil dal with tandoori chicken, steamed basmati rice, and a tomato salad
Turkey and Peach Salsa Wraps (see page 237)	A quarter of a melon	Penne pasta stir-fried with smoked salmon, olives, spinach, halved cherry tomatoes, garlic, and a little white wine
Pasta salad with corn, spring onion, pepper, cherry tomatoes, olives, and cucumber, and a little olive oil mayonnaise with sliced lean meat	Low-fat fruit yogurt	Fajitas made with lean beef or chicken and pepper. Serve with flour tortillas, salsa, guacamole, shredded lettuce, grated reduced-fat cheese, and natural yogurt
Pita bread with falafel, hummus, and tabbouleh	Carrot and celery sticks with tzatziki dip	Stir-fry with shrimp, veggies, and Hokkien noodles
Asian–style clear soup with noodles and seafood or chicken	A handful of cherries	Grilled or barbecued lamb kebabs served with chutney, spinach salad, and grilled pita bread slices
Open sandwich on toasted pumpernickel bread with ham, low-fat cream cheese, and salad veggies	A quarter of a melon	Grilled sardines with mixed-bean salsa (can of mixed beans, spring onion, fresh coriander, lemon juice, olives, olive oil, and halved cherry tomatoes) and a arugula salad
Roast lamb or beef with low-fat gravy and baked sweet potato, parsnip, beets, zucchini, and carrot	An apple	Bowl of vegetable and bean soup with whole-grain bread

WEEK 10

The drive to consume a certain volume of food each day is heavily ingrained in human behavior. We tend to consume the same physical bulk of food, regardless of its calorie content. Therefore, if the food we choose is energy dense—a little bit contains lots of calories (think cookies)—then it is very easy to eat too much. For this reason, it is critical to lower the energy density of our diet if we want to control our weight.

▶ FOOD GOAL
Lower the energy density of your diet.

▶ EXERCISE GOAL
Aim to walk for a total of 30 minutes on six days, at the same brisk pace as last week (around level 5 on the PRE scale) for the middle 15 minutes. *Plus* try to complete each of the resistance workouts, focusing on the upper and lower body respectively, three times during the week.

▶ ACTIVITY GOAL
Try out a new active hobby. For example, join a dancing class—ballroom, salsa, line dancing, Scottish dancing, or jazz; go rollerblading in the park; start golf lessons; or take your dog to agility classes.

▶ FOOD FOR THOUGHT
Incidental exercise—a lesson from the past.

▶ FOOD GOAL
Lower the energy density of your diet.

Reducing the energy density of your diet will help you reduce your energy intake and thereby facilitate weight loss. Energy density is a measure of how many calories are contained in a food. Foods with a high energy density contain a large number of calories in only a small amount of food. Chocolate is one example (22 calories per gram). Foods of low energy density provide few calories for a large quantity of food. Apples have a low energy density (2 calories per gram).

This week, we encourage you to examine the energy density of foods that you regularly eat, with the aim of reducing the overall energy density of your diet. If you haven't looked at it before, start taking a look at the nutrition information panel on foods and work out their energy density. To calculate energy density, divide the energy (calories) per 100 grams of the food by 100. A food can be considered energy dense if it has more than 5 calories per gram.

Sample nutrition information panel

Nutrient	Per 100 g
Energy (calories)	1,500
Protein (g)	9.5
Fat—total (g)	3.0
—saturated (g)	1.1
Carbohydrate (g)	72.2
—sugars (g)	5.4

This food has an energy density of 1,500 calories per 100 grams = 15 calories per gram. It has a high energy density.

Note that even though a food may be low in fat, it can still be high in energy density. High-fat foods will obviously be energy dense, but many commercial low-fat foods are high in energy density too. For example:

Energy density (calories/100 g) of some popular low-fat foods

Yogurt, low-fat, fruit	3
Bananas	4
Bread, white	10
Wheat biscuit breakfast cereal	14
Cornflakes	16
Pretzels	16
Rice crackers	17
Plain, sweet cookies	19

How to reduce the energy density of your diet

▶ Combine small servings of nutritious but energy-dense foods (such as nuts, cheese, and olive oil) with larger servings of less energy-dense foods (such as fruit, vegetables, pasta, rice, and grainy breads).

▶ Base meals on vegetables and legumes, using meat as an accompaniment and nuts as a condiment.

▶ Use oils (such as olive oil) where they will increase your enjoyment of less energy-dense foods (especially plant foods and fish) by improving the flavor of such dishes (for example, salads with dressing, roasted vegetables, and pan-fried fish). Added oils may also help your absorption of fat-soluble nutrients and phytochemicals from plant foods.

▶ Minimize foods containing hidden animal fats (fatty meat, full-fat dairy products, some fast/processed food) and hydrogenated plant fats (some fast/processed food, commercial cakes/cookies).

▶ Avoid eating large volumes of low-fat but energy-dense foods, particularly commercially processed cereals and cookies.

▶ Eat more fruit and vegetables. Large amounts of less energy-dense foods such as fruit and vegetables help to "dilute" the energy density of your diet.

—Add extra vegetables (frozen if you prefer) to stir-fried meat, chicken, shrimp, fish, or tofu.

—Eat salad daily.

—Include salad ingredients in sandwiches and rolls.

—Throw some veggies onto the barbecue with meat. Try zucchini, corn on the cob, peppers, mushrooms, eggplant, or thick slices of parboiled sweet potato or onion. (Use vegetable oil spray on a cold grill or a little olive oil to prevent sticking.)

—Try a vegetarian main dish at least once a week.

—For quick munching, keep celery, pepper, baby carrots, cucumber, broccoli, or cauliflower florets and cherry or grape tomatoes on hand.

■

TAKE CARE NOT TO *OVER*ESTIMATE HOW MUCH YOU DO OR *UNDER*ESTIMATE HOW MUCH YOU EAT.

■

▶ EXERCISE GOAL

Aim to walk for a total of 30 minutes on six days, at the same brisk pace as last week (around level 5 on the PRE scale) for the middle 15 minutes. *Plus* try to complete each of the resistance workouts, focusing on the upper and lower body respectively, three times during the week.

Resistance exercises

Workout 1	Lower-body exercises	"Core" strength abdominals and back
	Squats 1 set of 20	Full hover 2 x 30 seconds
	Squats with alternate leg extension 1 set of 20	Pointer 10 each side
	Lunges 10 each leg	
	Power lunges 20 alternate legs	
Workout 2	**Upper-body exercises**	
	Three-quarter push-ups 1 set of 20	Leg extensions 10 each leg
	Standing tricep extensions 1 set of 20	Ab curl 1 set of 20
	Bicep curl 1 set of 20	Oblique curl 20 each side

NEW EXERCISE

Squats with alternate leg extension

This advanced exercise really targets the bottom by adding a lift at the top of the squat. If possible, use a mirror to help you perfect your technique and avoid leaning to one side as you lift.

Strengthens and tones: legs and bottom

How to do it:
1. Perform your squat as before (see page 72), but as you rise, extend one leg at a 45-degree angle behind you, squeezing your bottom muscles as you do so.
2. Ensure that you maintain good posture by pulling in your navel and lifting your chest. Avoid swinging your leg—rather try for a controlled fluid movement without arching the back.
3. Repeat, lifting alternate legs each time.

How many: 20, using alternate legs each time

Sample journal

Monday	Tuesday	Wednesday	Thursday	Friday	Saturday	Sunday
30 min walk	30 min walk	30 min walk	30 min walk		30 min walk	30 min walk
+ workout 2	+ workout 1	+ workout 2	+ workout 1		+ workout 1	+ workout 2
40 min	40 min	40 min	40 min		40 min	40 min

▶ FOOD FOR THOUGHT
Incidental exercise—a lesson from the past.

Life today is far more challenging for our brains than it is for our bodies. Technology has made many of the everyday arduous tasks our grandparents would have done by hand far easier and less time-consuming. Washing machines, dishwashers, automatic car washes, drive-through restaurants, shopping malls, and the Internet all make life easier. The result, however, has been that modern life makes it very difficult for us to control our weight. Imagine living one day without any of this technology—washing your clothes or scrubbing the floor by hand, walking to the shops, walking home carrying heavy bags, chopping logs for the fire, creating everything you eat from raw ingredients, and washing up by hand.

Perhaps you still do some of these things, but imagine every day being filled with this level of activity. In addition to the higher levels of activity, food in the past was not so readily available or so appetizing —the wide choice of foods we have now encourages us to eat more. You can see that our environment works against our ability to control our weight. While no one wants to see a return to washing by hand and chopping wood for the fire, we can learn a lesson from the past and aim to become more active each and every day.

Consider your own lifestyle and environment and think about where you could build in a little more activity. It doesn't have to be much, and it probably won't feel like much at the time, but all those little movements will add up to a considerable increase in your energy output over the coming weeks, months, and years.

Some suggestions to build activity naturally into your days

At home

- Wash the car by hand.
- Iron while you watch television.
- Spend 20 minutes gardening.
- Mow the lawn.
- Clean one set of windows.
- Walk the dog.
- Stroll to your local shops.
- Spend an afternoon window shopping.
- Play with the kids.
- Vacuum the floor.

At work

- Use the printer down the hall or, even better, one floor up or down.
- Get up from your desk to speak with a colleague rather than using e-mail.
- Stand and stretch while on the telephone.
- Go outside at lunchtime for a stroll—walking while shopping counts!
- Use the upstairs or downstairs restroom.
- Volunteer to go out and buy the cappuccinos.
- Find an excuse to deliver something somewhere.
- Meeting with a colleague? Why not walk while you talk?

WEEK 10 MENU PLAN

	BREAKFAST	SNACK
MONDAY	Half a grapefruit followed by low-GI toast with avocado and sliced tomato	A handful of peanuts in their shell
TUESDAY	Natural muesli with sliced apple and low-fat milk	Oatmeal bread with hummus
WEDNESDAY	Carton of low-fat flavored milk and a banana	Slice of raisin toast with low-fat cream cheese
THURSDAY	Mixed-nut bar, an apple, and a low-fat yogurt	Oatmeal cookies and a skim-milk cappuccino
FRIDAY	Toasted whole-grain bread with ricotta cheese and fruit jam	A handful of red grapes
SATURDAY	Poached egg with smoked salmon, toasted sourdough, and spinach	A small glass of orange juice
SUNDAY	Low-fat yogurt with fruit salad and a sprinkle of mixed nuts and seeds	A glass of vegetable juice

LUNCH	SNACK	DINNER
Tuna Rice Paper Rolls (see page 238)	A nectarine	Chickpea and vegetable curry with steamed basmati rice
Bowl of vegetable soup with whole-grain crackers and low-fat cream cheese	A peach	Stir-fried greens with a grilled chicken breast and spiced lentils
Salad with a can of tuna, a handful of mixed beans, and a little yogurt dressing	Six raw Brazil nuts	Tortillas with refried beans, lettuce, salsa, chicken strips, and natural yogurt
Whole-grain bread with toasted reduced-fat cheese and tomato	An apple	Spinach and ricotta lasagna with a large green salad
Indian Chicken Burgers (see page 242) with hot chili salsa, warmed pita bread, and shredded lettuce	Natural yogurt with blueberries	Grilled lean steak with mashed sweet potato, steamed greens, and carrots
Whole-grain crackers with cottage cheese, cucumber, and sliced tomato and a cup of ready-to-serve soup	A handful of dried apricots	Asian–style noodle and seafood stir-fry with plenty of mixed veggies
Whole-grain sandwich with hard-boiled egg, olive oil mayonnaise, and salad	Fruit Parfaits (see page 262)	Roast chicken with baked veggies—sweet potato, beets, carrot, pumpkin, and squash. Drizzle with olive oil and balsamic vinegar and bake for 30 minutes.

WEEK 11

This week, focus on these goals:

▶ FOOD GOAL
Making the best of take-out food.

▶ EXERCISE GOAL
This week we split the walks into one shorter, brisker walk (30 minutes maintaining a brisk pace of level 5 for 20 minutes) and one longer but gentler walk (40 minutes at a steady pace of level 4). Aim to complete each walk three times. *Plus* try to complete the full resistance workout, incorporating both upper and lower body exercises, three times during the week.

▶ ACTIVITY GOAL
Whenever you are on a bus or a train for a short journey, choose to stand rather than sit.

▶ FOOD FOR THOUGHT
Can take-out food be part of a healthy diet?

▶ FOOD GOAL

Making the best of take-out food.

Who said take-out food can't be good for you? It definitely isn't if you eat it every night, but you can certainly put together a reasonable meal in minimal time with some astute choices and a little help from your local take-out provider. You will need to think about frequency, however, and that is one of the goals this week. How often is it reasonable for you or your family to be eating take-out foods for your main meal? Some would say once a month, others would say twice a week; we suggest no more than once or twice a week.

The other thing to think about is what you order. We'd like you to practice putting together a balanced meal with take-out food this week. Here are some examples using our three-step guide to planning a balanced meal.

Planning a balanced meal with take-out food

Low-GI carb	Fruit and vegetables	Protein and good fats
Home-cooked basmati rice	Stir-fry vegetables and cashew nuts	Braised beef
Basmati rice and lentil dal	Home-prepared green salad	Tandoori chicken
Corn on the cob	Home-made coleslaw with canola dressing	Barbecued chicken minus the skin

▶ EXERCISE GOAL

This week we split the walks into one shorter, brisker walk (30 minutes maintaining a brisk pace of level 5 for 20 minutes) and one longer but gentler walk (40 minutes at a steady pace of level 4). Aim to complete each walk three times. *Plus* try to complete the full resistance workout, incorporating both upper and lower body exercises, three times during the week.

Resistance exercises

This week we are going to combine the resistance training exercises into one effective workout to be undertaken three times a week. We suggest you do the workout on the days you complete your 30-minute walk to give you more time on the other three days for a longer walk. Maximizing your time in this way means that you never need to spend hours a day exercising, yet you continue to work toward your goals.

Lower-body exercises	
Squats	1 set of 20
Squats with alternate leg extension	1 set of 20
Lunges	10 each leg
Power lunges	20 alternating legs
Upper-body exercises	
Three-quarter push-ups	1 set of 20
Standing tricep extensions	1 set of 20
Bicep curl	1 set of 20
"Core" strength, abdominals and back	
Full hover	1 x 30 seconds
Pointer	10 each side
Leg extensions	10 each leg
Ab curl	1 set of 20
Oblique curl	20 each side

Sample journal

Monday	Tuesday	Wednesday	Thursday	Friday	Saturday	Sunday
40 min	30 min	40 min	30 min		40 min	30 min
walk 2	walk 1	walk 2	walk 1		walk 2	walk 1
	+ resistance workout		+ resistance workout			+ resistance workout
40 min	50 min	40 min	50 min		40 min	50 min

▶ FOOD FOR THOUGHT
Can take-out food be part of a healthy diet?

Most people eat take-out *sometimes*. That's okay; as we said before, it is the frequency that matters. The real problem exists for *some* people who eat take-out *most* of the time. With an average meal from a fast-food restaurant supplying about half of most people's daily energy requirements, those "two-for-one" or "super-size" meal deals, "free fries" and "delivered to your door" options really are better off resisted *most* of the time. So, decide on a reasonable, realistic limit for you and your family and stick to it.

On the plus side
- ▶ It's a welcome break from cooking.
- ▶ You can make "super-size" meals feed two adults or one adult and a child.
- ▶ Calorie-conscious items now appear on some menus.
- ▶ You can add something nutritious (such as a salad or vegetables) at home.

On the minus side
- ▶ The menu is often limited.
- ▶ Foods are high in calories, salt, and saturated fat.
- ▶ Meal deals that "upsize" for a small cost trap you into increasing your calorie intake.
- ▶ The difference between a small and a large can be double the calories.

- It takes so little time to eat the food from fast-food restaurants (no or little chewing required)—all those calories, and you don't even feel full.
- Even just a muffin and coffee can set you back 2,000 calories (a third of the day's requirement for some people).

For our suggestions on what to choose when ordering, see pages 184–90.

Here are some more healthy take-out options and quick-prep home alternatives:

- A regular hamburger with salad—hold the high-calorie extras such as cheese and bacon
- Salad sandwiches and rolls with ham, salmon, or egg included
- Vegetarian pizza (thin crust)—teamed with a tossed salad
- Take-out pasta with anything other than a creamy sauce
- Fish (lightly battered fillets) from the freezer—check for the varieties cooked in healthy oil—served with vegetables and salad
- Vegetarian lasagna
- Fresh noodles added to pre-cut stir-fry vegetable mix (fresh or frozen) with shrimp
- Canned refried beans on low-salt corn chips with dollops of avocado
- Chunks of skinless barbecued chicken added to a packet of chicken noodle soup with egg vermicelli, canned cream corn, frozen baby peas, and shallots to make a chicken and corn soup
- Vegetarian kebabs

WEEK 11 MENU PLAN

	BREAKFAST	SNACK
MONDAY	Grilled lean bacon served on a slice of toasted sourdough and topped with sliced tomato	A banana
TUESDAY	Toasted cheese-and-tomato sandwich from the take-out restaurant and an apple	A cup of cherries
WEDNESDAY	Toasted whole-grain bread topped with a little peanut butter and sliced banana	An apple
THURSDAY	Fruit salad with natural yogurt and a small handful of mixed nuts and seeds	A skim-milk cappuccino and oatmeal cookie
FRIDAY	On the run: a nut-and-seed bar and an apple	Low-fat fruit yogurt
SATURDAY	Scrambled egg with smoked salmon and spinach on a slice of toasted whole-grain bread	A pear
SUNDAY	Breakfast barley: cover the barley with water and simmer for 30–40 minutes until soft. Toward the end of cooking add a mixture of dried fruit, nuts, and seeds and serve with warmed low-fat milk.	An apple

LUNCH	SNACK	DINNER
Whole-grain roll with falafel, tabbouleh, and hummus	A nectarine	Lamb salad with tzatziki: grill or barbecue a lean lamb fillet and slice. Serve on a large salad of baby spinach leaves, semi-dried tomatoes, olives, cucumber, and peppers. Drizzle with tzatziki.
Mixed sushi box and miso soup	A small handful of raw almonds	Thai green chicken curry with a bag of Asian stir-fried frozen veggies added at home and served with home-cooked basmati rice
Multigrain bread sandwich with cream cheese, smoked salmon, and snow pea sprouts with salad	A low-fat fruit yogurt	Barbecued chicken, skin removed and meat chopped, added to a pot of chicken stock with long noodles, creamed corn, and shallots
Chicken noodle soup	Low-fat flavored milk	Mexican–style bean burrito with steamed basmati rice, salsa, and a green salad
Roast beef open sandwich on rye sourdough with plenty of salad veggies	A peach	Grilled fish fillet with a handful of chips, vinegar, and a watercress salad
Lentil, Beets, and Feta Salad (see page 240)	A handful of pistachios in their shells	Beef and vegetable stir-fry in black-bean sauce with Hokkien noodles
Sunday Roast with mashed sweet potato and steamed green peas, carrots, and Brussels sprouts	Creamed Rice with Rhubarb and Strawberries (see page 264)	Vegetable soup with melted cheese on toast

WEEK 12

You have made major changes over the last three months, and you should be enjoying the rewards of your efforts. Now is the time to start reinforcing all the changes you have made and making sure that none of your old habits are sneaking back in on a regular basis. Focus on the following goals this week:

▸ FOOD GOAL
Make healthy eating a habit.

▸ EXERCISE GOAL
As last week, aim to complete a shorter, brisker walk (30 minutes, maintaining a brisk pace of level 5 for 20 minutes) on three days, and one longer but gentler walk (40 minutes at a steady pace of level 4) on three days. *Plus* try to complete the full resistance workout, incorporating more advanced exercises for the upper and lower body, three times a week.

▸ ACTIVITY GOAL
Become an active person by nature, where you see every moment as an opportunity for movement. In other words, be the person who offers to run an errand, walk to the local shop for the papers, walk the dog, or carry the groceries home. Every moment of activity counts in the long run.

▸ FOOD FOR THOUGHT
Helping yourself toward healthier eating habits.

▶ FOOD GOAL
Make healthy eating a habit.

There is no magic bullet for permanent weight loss, but people who have lost weight and maintained it over the long haul reveal that weight-loss maintainers:

- ▶ Have a positive attitude toward changing their diet to improve health
- ▶ Possess a willingness to lose weight slowly
- ▶ Make lasting changes to their diet and exercise patterns
- ▶ Feel comfortable with, rather than restricted by, dietary changes

So how are you feeling about what you have done so far? It's time to reassess your eating habits with another food journal, to see how far you have come. As in Week 1, write down everything you eat and drink each day and compare it with the journal you kept at first. Hopefully, you will see some major differences. The aim is to keep it going! Remember, success is not about achieving a particular weight, but about changing the way you eat and live. It is the simple changes we make every day to the way we shop, cook, and eat that can change our lives.

■

MOTIVATION IS WHAT GETS YOU STARTED. HABIT IS WHAT KEEPS YOU GOING.

■

▶ EXERCISE GOAL
As last week, aim to complete a shorter, brisker walk (30 minutes, maintaining a brisk pace of level 5 for 20 minutes) on three days, and one longer but gentler walk (40 minutes at a steady pace of level 4) on three days. *Plus* try to complete the full resistance workout, incorporating more advanced exercises for the upper and lower body, three times during the week.

Resistance exercises

You should be feeling more energetic and alive, and starting to reap the rewards of all your efforts over the last weeks. This week, we make the resistance exercises a little more challenging to ensure your body keeps changing.

Lower-body exercises	
Squats	1 set of 20
Squats with alternate leg extension	1 set of 20
Lunges	10 each leg
Power lunges	20 alternating legs
Upper-body exercises	
Full push-ups	1 set of 10
Tricep push-ups	2 sets of 10
Bicep curl	1 set of 20
"Core" strength, abdominals and back	
Full hover	2 x 30 seconds
Pointer	10 each side
Leg extensions	10 each leg
Ab curl	1 set of 20
Oblique curl	20 each side

NEW EXERCISES

Full push-ups

Challenge yourself by increasing the load your body has to lift by performing your push-ups on your toes. As before, be sure to keep your bottom in line with your body (see pages 80 and 138).

How many: Try to complete 10 full push-ups, and then, if you need to, lower your knees to complete the second set of 10 in the kneeling position.

Tricep push-ups

This is a more challenging exercise for the triceps than the standing extensions, because your resistance in the push-up is coming from your own body weight, which is undoubtedly heavier than the weight you have been using.

Strengthens and tones: the back of the arm and the shoulder

How to do it:

1. From your regular three-quarter push-up position (see page 138), step your hands in closer until they are directly under your shoulders. You may find it more comfortable to make a fist rather than a flat hand as this allows you to keep your wrist straighter.
2. Lower your chest toward the floor and back, with your elbows tracking close to your rib cage.

How many: Try to complete 2 sets of 10 with a short rest in between

Sample diary

Monday	Tuesday	Wednesday	Thursday	Friday	Saturday	Sunday
40 min walk 2	30 min walk 1	40 min walk 2	30 min walk 1		40 min walk 2	30 min walk 1
	+ resistance workout		+ resistance workout			+ resistance workout
40 min	50 min	40 min	50 min		40 min	50 min

■

FIT PEOPLE BURN MORE FAT!

■

▶ FOOD FOR THOUGHT

Helping yourself toward healthier eating habits.

1. **Listen to your appetite.**
   The most normal way to eat is in response to your appetite. The first step for some people is simply tuning in to it, eating when they are hungry, and stopping when they feel full (not stuffed). It may help you to know that it's normal for your appetite to vary from day to day.

2. **Become aware of non-hungry eating.**

   Eating is an extremely complex behavior. There is a lot more to it than simply satisfying hunger or meeting nutrient needs. Food is part of socializing and celebrating, comforting and easing boredom. We eat food that is offered so as not to offend a host, we eat because we feel anxious or depressed, we finish off what the kids have left rather than waste it, we eat just because it looks good, or because it's there. All this non-hungry eating isn't wrong, but it can contribute to overeating and we need to be aware of it if we are to do anything about it.

3. **Eat regularly.**

   Have you ever noticed that the hungrier you are, the more tempting high-calorie foods such as chocolate, cookies, and chips are? And the harder it is to stop at one? You will find it easier to eat normally and control your appetite by regularly grazing on low-GI carbs.

4. **Think about what to eat, rather than what not to eat.**

   What happens if I ask you not to think of a pink elephant? You imagine it, right? The future is what we imagine, so rather than thinking of what you don't want to eat, think of what you do.

5. **Make overeating as difficult as possible.**

   When you go to have a slice of bread, take out one slice, then seal up the bag and put the loaf away. Put the spreads and toppings away before you sit down to eat. Out of sight generally means out of mind. Keep those occasional foods out of sight and, better still, don't buy them routinely.

6. **Make healthy foods more accessible.**

   Put healthy foods where you will find them first:

   - Washed, shiny apples and stone fruits (fruits with pits) in an attractive bowl in the fridge
   - Dried fruit and nuts in an airtight jar on your desk
   - Pre-sliced tomato and cucumber in the fridge, ready to use on sandwiches or crackers
   - Containers of low-fat yogurt in the fridge
   - A loaf of fruit bread by the toaster

These are just a few of the many ways you can increase your chances of eating the types of foods you planned to eat.

7. **Don't prepare enough to have leftovers.**
   If you cook too much and have leftovers, store them in containers and put them in the fridge before you sit down to eat the main meal. Still finding yourself tempted to go back for seconds? Try brushing your teeth soon after finishing a meal.

8. **Minimize distractions while you are eating.**
   Sitting in front of the television with a bag of chips or a chocolate bar, it is very easy to absentmindedly finish the whole thing. Focus on and savor what you are eating.

9. **Stick to regular times for your meals and snacks.**
   When you find yourself thinking about eating outside of your usual meal and snack times, try these four steps:

   - Delay.
   - Deep breathe.
   - Drink water.
   - Do something else.

10. **Put some thought and planning into your meals.**
    Preparing food is, for most of us, a necessity to eating, a fact of life. So take the time to cook—go to a class if you don't know how. Try different foods, write a shopping list, buy foods in season, get to know your local shopkeepers, shop regularly, and develop a passion for good, healthy food.

■

THINK ABOUT WHAT TO EAT
RATHER THAN WHAT NOT TO EAT.

■

WEEK 12 MENU PLAN

	BREAKFAST	**SNACK**
MONDAY	High-fiber cereal with sliced banana and low-fat milk	Fruit snack pack
TUESDAY	Toasted sourdough with avocado, smoked mackerel, and sliced tomato	Fruit salad
WEDNESDAY	Oatmeal with sliced banana, raisins, and low-fat milk	A slice of raisin toast with low-fat cream cheese
THURSDAY	High-protein cereal with sliced strawberries and low-fat milk	Oatmeal cookies
FRIDAY	Boiled eggs with whole-grain toast	An orange
SATURDAY	Half a grapefruit followed by whole-grain toast with reduced-fat cheese and sliced tomato	An apple
SUNDAY	Spinach and mushroom omelet with a slice of toasted soy-and-linseed bread	A glass of carrot-and-orange juice

LUNCH	SNACK	DINNER
Tuna sandwich on whole-grain bread with corn, olive oil mayonnaise, and sliced cucumber	Low-fat fruit yogurt	Mushroom and Vegetable Stir-fry (see page 246)
Lentil soup and a grainy roll	A handful of peanuts in their shell	Grilled lamb cutlets with sweet potato and pumpkin mash and steamed green beans, carrots, and broccoli
Ham and vegetable frittata	A handful of grapes	Chicken breast baked in orange juice served with boiled new potatoes and stir-fried greens
Tomato soup with whole-grain bread and low-fat cheese	A quarter of a melon	Beef Kebabs with Vegetable Noodle Salad (see page 248)
Chicken and salad tortilla wrap	A low-fat drinkable yogurt	Vegetable and chickpea curry with basmati rice
Ham, Corn, and Zucchini Muffins (see page 234) with salad	Carrot sticks with hummus dip	Cover a whole fish with chopped garlic, ginger, coriander leaves, and lemon juice and wrap in foil. Bake or barbe-cue for 30 minutes and serve with a large mixed salad.
Grilled sardines (canned or fresh) on sourdough toast and tomato and avocado salsa	An apple	Pork and vegetable stir-fry in oyster sauce with Hokkien noodles

PART THREE

Doing It for Life

Preventing Weight Gain

*A*re you familiar with the rhythm method of "girth" control? You gain some weight, lose it, gain some more, lose it—just like a yo-yo. Unfortunately, 95 percent of people who lose weight by "dieting" gain it all back again. And that is exactly the reason we have devoted this section to the topic of preventing weight gain.

In Doing It for Life, our focus turns from weight loss to weight maintenance, from "holding your hand" to giving you independence, in the form of the skills and knowledge that will maximize your chances of successful long-term weight control. Not only do we help you *entrench* a healthy new lifestyle, we also give you tried and tested tools, tips, and clever tricks for maintaining a healthy diet and keeping fit during different times in life—weekends, eating out, vacations, business travel, celebrations, and the ever-present emotional roller coaster. When facing these challenges, the more you know in advance, the better.

Just like the 12-week Action Plan, Doing It for Life has three themes that work in concert: meal planning, physical activity, and behavior modification. But it is your turn to take control and hold the reins. With practice and persistence—it will take about a year—you will find you have adopted a host of good habits and behaviors that are often unconscious and hard to break. Indeed, our aim is to have you well and truly hooked on the "high" that comes from living the healthy low-GI life.

Remember, success in the 12-week Action Plan should not be measured by the amount of weight or inches lost. What is more important is the extent to which your lifestyle has changed for the better, and the degree to which you have adhered to the eating and exercise guidelines.

Perhaps you lost 10 percent of your initial weight (that's terrific!), but remember, just 5 percent is a *significant* achievement that will markedly improve your health and vitality. We know some of you will want to lose even more weight, but it's important to spend at least the next three months maintaining your weight loss before tackling further weight loss by repeating the 12-week Action Plan. By using this alternating three-month pattern of weight loss and weight maintenance, you take the pressure off and give your body time to adjust.

In theory, maintaining your weight loss should be a lot easier than the process of losing it was. After all, at this stage of the game, the energy equation is balanced—that is to say, energy intake equals energy output. During weight loss, energy intake must be lower than energy output. So at this point you get to eat a little more than you have been eating during active weight loss. But beware, it's not the time to relax and let down your guard. And it is certainly not the time to stop exercising. If anything, this stage—preventing weight gain—is the most critical of all. It is going to take *at least twelve months* of persistent effort to convert your old eating and lifestyle pattern into a new and healthy one.

Unfortunately, many people mistakenly believe that once the desired amount of weight is lost, the hard part is over. Before they know it, they have regained the weight they lost, often in less time than it took to lose it—and with added "interest."

Why? There are several reasons why regaining weight is so easy. Research suggests that our bodies "remember" the previously higher weight and strive to attain it again. Hormones act to stimulate appetite and encourage excessive food intake. At your new weight, your body is also a smaller engine than it was in the past, so it requires less fuel to run. If you lost weight too rapidly and without exercising, then chances are you also lost excessive amounts of muscle, making your engine size even smaller.

Another reason why weight loss is so hard to maintain is that during dieting your resting metabolic rate (RMR), in absolute terms and on a per-pound basis, has dropped, often by as much as 10–12 percent. The RMR is nature's way of helping animals adapt to the environment in which they live. If food is scarce, your body will get by with less fuel by reducing the engine revs. One *proven* benefit of the Low GI Diet Revolution is that the reduction in RMR that comes with the weight loss is much smaller than on other diets, around 5 percent, instead of 10 percent. The Low GI Diet Revolution leads to less fluctuation in blood-glucose levels, and consequently your body regulates fuel better, with no shortage of either glucose or fat to burn at any time.

Whatever the reason for the decline in energy expenditure, the bottom line is that you need to remain focused on eating well and exercising regularly. If you drift back into your old eating habits and couch potato lifestyle, then the writing's on the wall. Importantly, your healthy low-GI diet will be easy to maintain, because, unlike low-carb or calorie-restricted diets, it is not an enormous departure from the individual norm. Concentrating on the *quality*, rather than *quantity*, of carbs and fats gives you built-in flexibility and freedom.

Characteristics of long-term "weight losers"

They engage in high levels of physical activity.
Their exercise is usually brisk walking but often includes weight lifting.
They use a pedometer to count steps per day (see pages 210–12).
They watch the total amount of food eaten.
They eat a reduced-fat, not low-carb, diet.
They frequently "self-monitor" (use diet and activity journals).

Characteristics of those who regain weight

They resume their old ways.
They relax their dietary restraint.
They reduce their physical activity.

■

BE A FULL-TIME WEIGHT MAINTAINER, NOT A PART-TIME LOSER.

■

PLANNING THE RIGHT MEALS FOR WEIGHT MAINTENANCE

It's time to see if you can swim without the floaties. In the 12-week Action Plan, we did all the meal planning for you. It is your turn now to plan your own healthy low-GI meals. The good news is that because you aren't trying to *lose* more weight, you can eat a little more each day. This could be an extra serving of fruit or of a low-fat dairy food, or both if you weigh more than 220 pounds. You might even like to have an extra indulgence occasionally. Although the goal at this stage is to maintain your current weight, it's still necessary to be choosy about your food. This means not straying too far from the Low GI Diet Revolution guidelines (pages 38–52). You can include treat foods once a day, but it's absolutely critical that you meet your exercise and activity goals.

> Here's a hot tip—adding an extra serving of protein to your day in the form of lean meat, fish, or chicken is especially helpful in preventing weight gain. New studies are showing that adding 1 to 2 ounces protein to the diet helps people maintain weight loss in the long term. This equates to about 7 ounces (raw weight) of lean steak, poultry, or fish. The reason? Turn back to page 103, where we summarized protein's magic.

If you are finding your weight loss difficult to maintain, you probably need to revise your serving sizes. You could be eating healthy foods but are simply eating too much of some. In the past twenty years, the typical serving size of foods has increased markedly. This is most obvious in the restaurant and fast-food industry, where providing "value" for money—more food for fewer dollars—is a common marketing approach (see the following box overleaf). Energy-dense, calorie-laden food has become more readily available for relatively little extra cost. This is not good news for weight control.

Average serving sizes are on the rise

	1980	2000
Soft drink	12 ounces	16 ounces
Chips	1 ounce	1¾ ounce
French fries	5¼ ounces	9 ounces
Popcorn	2 cups	4 cups

Babies and young children subconsciously "listen" to their natural body signals to eat when they are hungry and to stop when they are satisfied. Many adults (and older children) have lost touch with this fundamental physiological regulation of food intake. Consequently, in an environment of highly appetizing, constantly visible, energy-dense food, it's just too easy to overeat. Instead of relying on our bodies' natural signals of hunger and satiety to decide how much to eat, we use environmental and learned behavioral cues, such as finishing all that's on our plate (it's wasting food not to!) or eating all that's offered (seconds, anyone?).

■

LISTEN TO YOUR APPETITE AND LET IT GUIDE HOW MUCH YOU EAT.

■

Here are a few tips for keeping your food intake in line with your bodily requirements. First, revisit some of the behavioral techniques listed in Week 12 (see pages 163–65) of the Action Plan. Listen to your body's cues for food intake and fine-tune your eating behavior. Second, ensure that you are eating foods in the correct proportions using our three-step guide to meal planning:

1. **Start** with a low GI carbohydrate.
2. **Add** a generous serving of vegetables or fruit.
3. **Plus** add some protein with a little healthy fat for good measure.

On the next page we give examples of how to build your meals around low-GI carbs.

Make breakfast a priority

Your mother was right—breakfast really is the most important meal of the day. It's particularly important for weight control, not only because it recharges your brain, but because it speeds up your metabolism after an overnight "fast."

Those who eat the biggest breakfasts eat *fewer* calories over the whole day. Why? It is possible that a prolonged interval between dinner and the next meal triggers counter-regulatory hormones that increase eating behavior. Furthermore, the longer you maintain your "fast" or delay breakfast, the more insulin-resistant you become. This means that whatever you eat next will produce an elevated insulin response, driving greater carbohydrate oxidation and reducing the burning of fat. All of the people on the National Weight Control Registry (a registry of people who have lost at least 30 pounds and kept it off for at least twelve months) were found to be having breakfast on most days of the week. You can study their habits more closely by visiting the Web site at www.nwcr.ws.

Breakfasts

Low-GI carb	+	Fruit and vegetables	+	Protein and good fat	=	Balanced low-GI meal
Muesli and yogurt		Strawberries and yogurt		Low-fat milk		Muesli with fruit
Baked beans		Mushrooms		Poached egg		Poached eggs, mushrooms, and baked beans
Rolled oats		Raisins with banana slices		Low-fat milk		Raisin and banana oatmeal
Whole-grain toast		Fresh, ripe, sliced tomato and lettuce		Sliced bacon and a smear of barbecue sauce		BLT sandwich
Low-fat plain yogurt with a drizzle of honey		Mashed ripe banana		Low-fat milk with a dash of nutmeg		Banana smoothie
Sourdough toast		Tomato juice		Herrings with a squeeze of lemon		Herrings on sourdough
Whole-grain toast		Sliced red apple		Reduced-fat cheddar cheese		Toasted cheese-and-apple sandwiches
Low-fat vanilla yogurt		Fresh chopped seasonal fruit		Mixed nuts and seeds		Fruit and nut yogurt
Fruit toast		Fruit spread or fresh sliced stone fruit		Fresh ricotta cheese		Raisin toast with ricotta and fruit
Whole-grain toast		Shallots, mushrooms, tomatoes, and parsley		Eggs and grated reduced-fat cheese		Savory omelet on toast

Light Meals

Low-GI + carb	Fruit and + vegetables	Protein and = good fat	Balanced low-GI meal
Sourdough bread	Lettuce, tomato, beets, onion	Minute steak	Steak sandwich
Flat bread	Tabbouleh salad, hummus	Falafel and kebab	Falafel roll
Sweet corn on the cob	Coleslaw	Barbecued chicken	Chicken and salad
Whole-grain bread	Lettuce, tomato, cucumber, beets, alfalfa, grated carrot, and onion	Shaved ham	Ham sandwich and salad
Pasta	Napoletana sauce	Shaved parmesan cheese	Pasta Napoletana
Whole-grain bread	Sliced ripe tomatoes drizzled with olive oil and balsamic vinegar plus torn basil	Canned tuna (drained) combined with garlic, capers, parsley, and olive oil, plus a little hummus to spread on the bread	Tuna tapenade and tomato salad
Mixed-grain bread	Lettuce, cucumber, and white onion	Red salmon, plus a little light cream cheese to spread on the bread	Salmon and lettuce sandwich
Toasted sourdough rubbed with a clove of garlic	Slow-roasted tomatoes and field mushrooms	Baked ricotta with herbed olive oil for dressing	Garlic toast with tomatoes, mushrooms, and baked ricotta
Five-bean mix with diced pepper and shallots, tossed in oil, lemon, and parsley	Salad greens, tomato, grated carrot, and diced cucumber	Grated cheddar cheese	Cheese and bean salad

Main Meals

Low-GI carb	+ Fruit and vegetables	+ Protein and good fat	= Balanced low-GI meal
Corn tortilla with refried beans	Shredded lettuce, tomato, diced celery, and cucumber with tomato salsa	Lean ground beef, grated cheese, and a dollop of mayonnaise for the salad	Beef and bean tortillas with salad
Canned brown lentils	Diced tomato, shredded English spinach, and lemon juice	Lamb fillet marinated in olive oil, garlic, and oregano	Barbecued Lamb with Lentil Salad and Yogurt Dressing (see page 250)
Sweet potato	A bunch of aruglua or mixed salad greens	Fillets of bream, ocean perch, flake, or ling brushed with olive oil and black pepper	Sweet Potato Fish cakes (see page 241)
Basmati rice and dal	Curry powder or paste plus cauliflower, carrot, green peas, and canned tomatoes	Diced beef or lamb browned in canola oil with garlic and onion	Indian curry and rice
Baby new potatoes steamed and cooled	Fresh green beans, (blanched), cherry tomatoes (halved) and kalamata olives, dressed with olive oil and red wine vinegar	Canned tuna in water (drained) and hard-boiled egg (quartered)	Tuna salad
Sweet potato	Strips of red pepper and red onion plus steamed green beans	Eggs	Vegetable Frittata (see page 232) with green beans
Canned borlotti beans	Canned tomatoes, onions, garlic, carrots, celery, and rutabaga	Lean ground beef browned in olive oil	Beef and bean casserole
Steamed basmati rice	Asian stir-fry frozen vegetable mix or fresh snow peas, baby corn, carrot, onion, and Asian greens	Chicken, beef, lamb, or pork strips stir-fried in peanut oil with chili plum sauce	Stir-fry with rice
Steamed corn on the cob	Mixed salad	Skinless barbecued chicken	Chicken with salad
Spaghetti	Onion, garlic, mushrooms, and pepper with a jar of tomato pasta sauce	Lean ground beef	Spaghetti Bolognese

ONE MEAL FOR THE WHOLE FAMILY

Our readers and clients often tell us that one of the side benefits of eating better is that their partner or family is doing so, too. Sometimes it seems as if the others were just waiting for someone to take the lead. What does this tell us about trying to lose weight? Family support is a vital part of eating and living well. If one person in a household changes his or her eating habits, the whole household may have to adapt. All the more reason to steer clear of untested fad diets. Here are some tips for harmonious family eating.

Aim to prepare the same meal for the whole family

Separate meals will only serve to alienate the person who is trying to change. If there is a diversity of tastes within the family, prepare a range of foods and allow them to serve themselves at the table.

The Ten Commandments of maintaining weight loss

1. Never skip meals (or you will reduce your metabolic rate).
2. Eat a really good breakfast.
3. Eat at least three to four times a day.
4. Limit television to less than 12 hours per week.
5. Choose low-GI carbs at every meal.
6. Eat lean protein sources at every meal.
7. Don't skimp on the fats—just choose healthy ones.
8. Eat seven servings of fruit and veggies every day.
9. Schedule moderate physical activity for 30–60 minutes on six days out of seven.
10. On the seventh day, relax.

Eat dinner together

As we all know, there is something uniting about sharing a meal together. Think about making meals special with extra touches such as using your favorite china, lighting candles, having flowers on the table, or putting on some background music. Eating together will also improve the quality of your children's diet. Kids who eat with their families on most days have significantly better nutrient intakes and are far more likely to eat the recommended amounts of fruit and vegetables; their diets also contain less saturated fat and have a lower GI than those of children who don't.

Turning off the television and having dinner-table conversations are some of the best things you can do for your kids' intellectual development.

Growing good food habits in your children

1. Don't restrict their calories.

2. Serve sensible portions (about the size of the child's fist).

3. Allow all foods, including desserts.

4. Involve them in shopping and in food preparation.

5. Make a general rule: three bites of every type of food on the plate.

6. Limit soft drinks and fruit juices; replace with low-fat milk.

7. Don't keep soft drinks in the house; purchase them only outside the home.

8. Limit fast food to twice per week.

Involve others in food choices and meal planning

Talk about it with one another. Ask, "What are the most important foods to you?" "Which type of low-fat milk would you like to try?" or "Here's a list of recommended snacks, which would you prefer?"

Make family lifestyle changes

For example, take a stroll together after dinner, have a television-free night once a week, or try having meals outdoors.

Don't buy food you want to avoid

If your kids are clamoring for foods that you are trying to avoid, give them the money that you would normally spend on those treats. Let them decide what they want to buy with it.

Enjoy special treats together when the occasion arises

Food is a traditional part of most celebrations, and treats will be even more special if you reserve them for these times.

EAT WELL ON WEEKENDS AND VACATIONS

Do you manage to maintain healthy eating habits diligently through the week but let things slide when you get to the weekend? Or have you been holding out for vacation to indulge in your favorite snack foods, take-out, bakeries, and restaurants? The problem with this approach is that it can be difficult to resume your hard-earned good habits after the break. While it's good to have one day free of restrictions and obligations, any longer makes it likely you will slip back into old, familiar ways. So instead of denying yourself your favorite meal, enjoy it once a week, whatever the occasion, and approach vacations and weekends as an extension of your new, healthier lifestyle.

One of the hardest places to make healthy choices is on the road. It might seem easy to pull into the drive-thru for a bite to eat, but you will save money if you plan a proper stop. Choose from the menu sensibly and enjoy the break from routine. Alternatively, if you know there is a rest stop or scenic spot en route, plan ahead and enjoy a roadside picnic. A lookout, walking track, or park can give you the opportunity not only to refuel your batteries, but to stretch those legs and breathe in some fresh air to help break up the drive. Pack some sandwiches (individually wrapped and packed in a plastic container so they don't get squashed) and some easy-to-eat fruit such as apples, bananas, or grapes. Some icy bottled water is also a good idea, especially during the summer.

A self-catered vacation—in an apartment or vacation home—will give you far more control over your food choices, but, understandably, you won't want to spend all your time preparing food! So make it easy with a little forethought and preparation. Consider taking an appliance you can use for quick meals, such as a sandwich maker or portable grill. Or take the blender to make smoothies for breakfast or for a delicious snack. If there will be lots of sitting around, perhaps you could take that popcorn maker or vegetable juicer that never gets much use. Kebab skewers and barbecue tools can be very handy, too.

If you are self-catering, you might take all the food with you or plan a trip to the supermarket when you first arrive. You will find it easier if you have thought of some easy meals beforehand and written yourself a shopping list.

Meals to make anywhere

▶ Make a home-made pizza from pita bread spread with cheese and toppings.

▶ Combine a can of tuna, chopped tomatoes, and some antipasto vegetables for an easy pasta sauce.

▶ Burritos can be made out of avocado, tortillas, and a can of refried beans.

Snacks to have on hand when you're away from home

▶ Fresh fruit—try some locally grown produce

▶ Unsalted nuts and dried fruit

▶ A low-saturated-fat dip such as hummus or mashed avocado, scooped up with carrot sticks and celery

▶ Low-fat fruit yogurts

Simple barbecue meals

A barbecue is an easy, popular meal while you're out and about or away on vacation.

▶ Try pieces of marinated lean steak or shrimp.

▶ Add some vegetables to the barbecue: mushrooms, halved tomatoes, sliced potato, corn on the cob (in its husk), pineapple, peppers, and onions.

▶ For dessert, try barbecued bananas in their skin (for a treat, add some chocolate hazelnut spread!).

▶ A prepared salad such as coleslaw or tabbouleh can be purchased, or make your own combination of fresh salad vegetables and add the dressing just before serving.

> **Tip:** If you are unsure if you will find a barbecue, or if there are fire restrictions in place, just take along a barbecued chicken.

Plan a picnic

Whether you are out on a day trip, feeding a horde of kids, or just looking for something different to offer friends, pack it all up in a basket and head for the great outdoors. You will enjoy the break from routine and expend some energy in the process.

Here are some tasty ideas:

- Olives, marinated mushrooms, peppers, and eggplant, semi-dried tomatoes, and a home-made pasta salad
- Vegetable frittata, a handful of salad greens, and tiny new potatoes with vinegar and mint
- Lean cold meats such as turkey breast, ham, pastrami, or marinated chicken drumsticks
- Smoked trout or salmon, fresh oysters, or shrimp
- Tabbouleh, hummus, pita bread, and thin slices of tender roast lamb with a chickpea or lentil salad
- Fresh fruits, such as grapes, sliced mango, and strawberries
- A piece of good cheese and fresh sourdough bread
- Cool mineral or soda water with a twist of lime or lemon

Day-trip survival kit

Besides taking along items such as sunscreen and insect repellent, pack up an insulated bag or a cooler with this collection:

- Cold bottled water
- Fresh sandwiches with easy, simple fillings such as sliced cheese and pickle, ham and mustard, and turkey breast with cranberry jelly
- Washed and dried fresh fruit, such as small crisp apples or grapes

EATING OUT THE LOW-GI WAY

Whether you think it is compatible with healthy eating or not, statistics tell us that at some point soon you are going to be eating out or buying take-out food. Eating out can really test your resolve as far as healthy eating goes. And as with any food choice, the more often we eat out, the more important it is that we choose healthy options. If you eat out only once a month you needn't be too fussy, but if it's three to four times a week, good choices are critical. Here are our survival tips to help you when you're eating out.

Don't go ravenously hungry

If you are planning a big night out, don't starve yourself through the day. All that does is reduce your metabolic rate. Eat a light breakfast and lunch, and before you go, have a quick snack—try a slice of grainy bread. This takes the edge off your appetite and you will be less likely to overeat.

Take an extra walk

When you know you will be eating and drinking more than usual, get some extra exercise, preferably beforehand. If it is feasible, walk to the restaurant. At the very least, try not to park right outside the restaurant.

Before you order

Ask for water as soon as you arrive and guzzle some down before your meal. It will begin filling your stomach immediately.

Bypass the bread

Send the bread basket away (unless it is exceptional or low-GI bread).

Remember 1, 2, 3

No, we are not talking about three-course meals, but the three basic parts to a healthy, balanced meal:

1. Low-GI carbs
2. Vegetables or salad
3. Protein—meat, seafood, poultry, or a vegetarian alternative such as tofu

Ensure that what you order provides all three parts.

Keep it simple

Often simple fare is the healthiest. You know where you stand with green salad, oysters au naturel, steak, roast lamb, or a fresh fruit plate.

Halve it

Order an appetizer for your main course or specify appetizer size. Alternatively, eat *only half* of everything on your plate.

Hold the fries

Tell the waiter to hold the fries. In some restaurants, french fries or chips come with the meal whether you order them or not. Their high energy density, high GI value, and high saturated-fat content make them weight-control enemy number one.

Pace yourself

Never order all courses at once. Try ordering one at a time and then see how you feel before ordering the next course. This gives the receptors in your stomach time to send a satiety signal to your brain.

Save sauce for the side

Ask for the sauce separately. There are lots of advantages to doing this. Number one: if it is not to your taste, you haven't spoiled your entire meal. Number two: you might end up getting more real food on your plate—such as more shrimp in your salad. And, of course, if the sauce is terribly fatty or oily, at least you can control the amount you eat.

Take your time

Relax and enjoy the food that is being prepared *for* you, not *by* you.

If you don't want it, leave it

It's okay to leave some food on your plate. If you don't want to go home feeling like a stuffed walrus, put your knife and fork down as soon as you feel comfortably satisfied.

Be discerning with drinks

Make water your first choice. Ask for some routinely, whether you feel like drinking it or not. Chances are you will drink it if it is in front of you. Go easy on the sugary drinks, because they tend to bypass satiety mechanisms. Drink no more than one to three glasses of alcohol. Remember, alcohol has almost twice as much energy as carbohydrate.

Spoons for two

The Low GI Diet Revolution is not about deprivation, so if you really feel like it, go ahead and have a dessert; but why not share it with someone?

Walk it off

After a restaurant meal, walk home or back to the office and climb the stairs rather than using the elevator.

Finding the low-GI choice on the menu

Indian food

The traditional accompaniment for Indian dishes is steamed basmati rice, which is a classic low-GI choice. Lentil dal offers another low-GI accompaniment, but make sure they don't add the oil topping (*tadka*).

Unleavened breads such as chapati or roti may have lower GI values than normal bread, but they will boost the carbohydrate content of the meal and increase the GL.

Our suggestions:
- *Tikka* (dry roasted) or tandoori (marinated in spices and yogurt) chicken
- Basmati rice
- Cucumber *raita*
- Spicy spinach (*saag*)

Japanese food

Japanese sushi rice has a low GI, and any refrigerated rice has a lower GI than when it is freshly cooked. The vinegar used in the preparation of sushi helps keep the GI low (acidity helps slow stomach emptying), and so do the viscous fibers in the seaweed. Typical ingredients and flavors to enjoy are *shoyu* (Japanese soy sauce), *mirin* (rice wine), wasabi (a strong horseradish), miso (soybean paste), pickled ginger (*oshinko*), sesame seeds, and sesame oil. Go easy on deep-fried dishes such as tempura.

Japanese restaurants are great places to stock up on omega-3 fats, since dishes such as sushi and sashimi made with salmon and tuna contain high amounts of beneficial polyunsaturated fatty acids.

Our suggestions:
- Miso soup
- Sushi
- Teppanyaki (steak, seafood, and vegetables)

- Yakitori (skewered chicken and onions in teriyaki sauce)
- Sashimi (thinly sliced raw fish or beef)
- Shabu-shabu (thin slices of beef quickly cooked with mushrooms, cabbage, and other vegetables)
- Side orders such as seaweed salad, wasabi, soy sauce, and pickled ginger

Thai food

Thai food is generally sweet and spicy and contains aromatic ingredients such as basil, lemongrass, and galangal. Spicy Thai salads, which usually contain seafood, chicken, or meat, are a delicious light meal. For starters, avoid the deep-fried items such as spring rolls.

One downside to Thai cuisine is the coconut milk, which really raises the saturated fat content of Thai curry. So don't feel you have to consume all of the sauce or soup. The traditional accompaniment to Thai food is plain, steamed Jasmine rice, but this has a very high GI value, so you are better off if you can reduce the quantity. Noodles are always on the menu as well, but avoid fried versions. Boiled rice noodles may be an option. Limit yourself to a small helping, or, if you are having take-out, you could cook up some basmati rice at home as an accompaniment.

Our suggestions:
- Tom yam—hot and sour soup
- Thai beef or chicken salad
- Wok-tossed meats or seafood
- Stir-fried mixed vegetables
- Small serving of steamed noodles or rice
- Fresh spring rolls (not fried)

Italian food

The big plus with Italian restaurants is the plentiful supply of low-GI pasta with an array of sauces. Good choices are *arrabiata*, puttanesca, Napoletana, and marinara sauces (without cream). Despite what you may think, most Italians don't sit down to huge bowls of pasta, so don't be afraid to leave some on your plate (or order an appetizer size). The GI may be low, but a large serving of pasta will have a high GL. Other good choices include minestrone and vegetable dishes, lean veal, and grilled seafood. Steer clear of crumbed and deep-fried seafood.

Our suggestions:
- Minestrone soup
- Veal scallopini in tomato-based sauce
- Prosciutto (paper-thin slices of Italian ham) wrapped around melon
- Barbecued or grilled seafood such as calamari or octopus
- Roasted or grilled fillet of beef, lamb loin, or poultry
- Green garden salad with olive oil and balsamic vinegar
- Sorbet, gelato, or a fresh fruit platter
- Appetizer-size pasta with seafood and tomato or stock-based sauce

---

Tips for those who routinely eat in restaurants

1. *Walk* to the restaurant if possible.

2. Order water as soon as you arrive.

3. Send the bread basket away (unless it's exceptional).

4. Order green salad, oysters au naturel, or soup for an appetizer.

5. Order an appetizer for your main course (or specify appetizer size).

6. Alternatively, eat only half of everything on your plate.

7. Tell the waiter to hold the french fries.

8. Share dessert with a dining companion.

9. Drink no more than one to three glasses of alcohol.

10. Walk back to your destination or climb the stairs.

Greek and Middle Eastern food

In Mediterranean cuisine, olive oil, lemon, garlic, and onions and other vegetables abound. Many dishes are grilled, and specialties such as barbecued octopus or grilled sardines are excellent choices. You will find regular bread replaced with flat bread or Turkish bread, while potatoes are replaced with whole grains such as bulgur (in tabbouleh) and couscous.

Among the small appetizing meze dishes, you may pick and choose what you like. Many of the choices are healthy, including hummus, baba ghanoush, olives, tzatziki, and dolmades.

Our suggestions:
- Meze platter with pita bread
- Souvlaki (grilled skewers of meat with vegetables)
- Kofta (balls of ground lamb with bulgur wheat)
- Greek salad of fresh lettuce, tomato, olives, feta, and pepper, with balsamic dressing or oil and lemon
- Fresh fruit platter
- Falafel with tabbouleh and hummus with a flat bread

STAYING ON TRACK WHILE TRAVELING FOR BUSINESS

Whether you love it or hate it, regular business travel necessitates some thought and planning to avoid disrupting your healthy lifestyle routine.

Breakfast

There is no reason why breakfast away from home shouldn't be as good, if not better, than what you normally have. You may even have more time on your hands to enjoy it. A buffet breakfast can be a great place to sample some different breakfast foods from around the world. The biggest hazard is overeating—because it's all there in front of you, it's easy to take more than you need. Good options include:

- Fruit—fresh fruit or juice is always available, and this is a great way to boost your daily fruit intake. Try a fruit you've never had before with yogurt on top.
- Cereal with low-fat milk—dry cereals should be selected with care. Muesli, fruit, and yogurt are more sustaining options.
- Cooked breakfast—go with the grainy bread for toast, skip the butter or margarine, and top it with poached or scrambled eggs. This gives you protein without too many calories and can make the whole meal more sustaining. Side orders such as mushrooms and tomato add micronutrients without excessive calories.

Lunch

Lunch these days is mostly a light affair, but if it isn't, try to make your evening meal light. By light we mean big on salad and vegetables. In fact, it's vital to include vegetables with lunch if you are to meet the daily recommendation of at least five servings a day. Add protein for sustenance, but don't go heavy on high-GI carbs at lunch if you want to minimize a post-lunch dip in energy levels. If you are on the go, stop at a suitable place that sells grainy bread, salad mixes, and fresh fruit.

Dinner

Take a look at our recommendations on pages 184–90 for good choices when you are eating out. Stick with simple options for dinner—grilled steak, chicken breast, fish or seafood with vegetables or salad. While ordering, think about how much energy you have used during the day, and order to match.

Snacks

For a start, empty the minibar and stock it with a couple of low-fat yogurts and a few bananas or apples. Another solution is to prepare snacks in advance and take enough to last you through the trip. Dried fruit and nuts make nutritious lightweight snacks.

Activity tip

While away on business, confined to hotel rooms and meeting rooms, it can be hard to find any time for activity. We suggest you pack a jump rope and find 15 minutes a day to exercise in your hotel room. Alternatively, if the stairs are accessible and safe, ask for a room on the second or third floor and use them as you come and go.

STRESS EATING—CAN YOU COPE?

Are you a stress eater—someone who raids the cookie jar or the freezer when the going gets tough, the deadlines loom, and the obligations mount? When you are disappointed in something or someone, or grieving the loss of anything, does food help fill the void? Afterward you feel let down, guilty, more stressed, and the cycle begins to repeat itself. Does this pattern sound familiar?

You are not alone. About 50 percent of people feel hungry when stressed, and women struggle with this problem more than men. And it's not just a failure of willpower—it's a question of hormones. Science can now explain the phenomenon of "emotional" eating. When we are in immediate physical danger, the hormone cortisol is flushed into the bloodstream as part of the fight-or-flight response. A less marked but prolonged rise occurs when we are simply under pressure to perform—in other words, stressed. Cortisol's function is to help us cope with the challenge by mobilizing fuels (glucose and fat) for exceptional physical performance. Another action of cortisol is to increase our appetite—after all, eating will provide more fuel for meeting the next challenge.

This direct connection between cortisol and hunger spells trouble, especially if you're dieting. Dieters have cortisol levels about 20 percent higher than less restrained eaters. The constant challenge to restrict energy intake is a cause of stress in itself. Researchers at Yale University found that women with the highest levels of cortisol ate double the amount of energy-dense food (think doughnuts or chocolate) than those with low cortisol levels. Furthermore, stress actually makes those foods taste better, enhancing the flavor of sweet, fatty foods.

Cortisol's actions would have been entirely appropriate in the past, when we ran for our lives as hunter-gatherers, when fear of wild animals was a constant threat. But these days the challenges we face are mental rather than physical, and we don't need all those extra calories to perform cognitive feats. The difficulty today in our rush-rush world is that we often feel under constant pressure. Indeed, in one survey, nearly 30 percent of people admitted that they have a "red alert" day almost daily. It's no coincidence that the increase in overweight people is matched with rising rates of stress—the two are linked physiologically.

One of cortisol's downstream effects is to increase insulin levels and thereby promote fat storage around the waist rather than elsewhere. That is because fat around the stomach is easy to convert to instant energy compared with fat that is stored in the thighs or just under the skin. Fat stored in the belly is "emergency" energy. Even some thin women with high cortisol levels have been found to have a potbelly. Unfortunately, you won't be drawing on that emergency supply when your mind, not your legs, is doing the running. If both cortisol and insulin stay high for several hours, they drive glucose burning instead of fat burning.

How to pull yourself together

You guessed it—exercise! Not just because it burns excess energy, but also because it releases the "feel-good" chemicals that negate anxiety and stress. A quick bout of exercise can even stop a surge in cortisol and reduce food cravings in their tracks. For example, if you are in the office, a quick run up the stairs may be all it takes to blunt the cortisol spike.

Stopping stress in its tracks

Step 1: Recognize that stress, anxiety, and worry make you hungry.

Step 2: Recognize that there's a physical reason behind it.

Step 3: Give in to the hunger, but make it a low-GI, high-protein snack (see suggestions below).

Step 4: Get on your bike or into your sneakers and move it.

Step 5: Increase your heart rate until it's really pumping for at least 20 minutes.

Step 6: Afterward, savor the feeling of invigoration that only exercise can give.

Cortisol emergency fixes

apple slices with peanut butter

strawberries dipped in chocolate-hazelnut spread

a sweet yogurt topped with berries

a good cheese with celery sticks

a handful almonds and muscatel raisins

a handful of chocolate-covered raisins

a cookie or two if that's what it takes

■

A FALL IN CORTISOL MEANS A WORLD OF DIFFERENCE IN ATTITUDE AND A MORE PRODUCTIVE YOU.

■

Apart from exercise, there are a few other simple tricks to deal more effectively with stress on a long-term basis:

1. Listen to music while you work.
2. Keep a serene or smiling Buddha on your desktop.
3. Listen to a relaxation tape while driving to and from work.
4. Connect with a good friend or group of friends.
5. Take a yoga class.
6. Get a massage.
7. Take a bath.
8. Get seven to eight hours' sleep (the sleep-deprived have higher cortisol levels).

ALL-NIGHT EATERS

"Night eating syndrome" was first reported fifty years ago, but scientists are now taking a new look at it. Only 1 to 2 percent of the population is thought to suffer from some of the symptoms of this condition, but it is more common among overweight people, and the occurrence may be as high as one in four among obese individuals.

In recent studies at the University of Pennsylvania, sufferers were monitored in sleep laboratories and compared with matched-for-weight "control" subjects who did not report night eating. Characteristically, the signs and symptoms of the all-night eaters were:

- Little or no appetite for breakfast
- First meal delayed for several hours after waking
- Increased appetite at night
- Eating more in the evening
- Consuming more than half of the daily energy intake after 8 PM
- Trouble falling asleep or staying asleep (insomnia)
- Waking frequently (more than one to two times a night) and then eating
- Feeling tense, anxious, or guilty while eating
- Tending to eat carb-rich foods (sugars, starches)

The preferred snack of the night eaters studied was a peanut butter sandwich (about 360 calories, with carbohydrate as the dominant
energy source). They remembered what they ate, unlike people with
the rare nighttime eating disorder linked to sleepwalking. In contrast
to binge eaters, who have short, intense bursts of eating, night eaters
eat continuously throughout the evening and night. They do not purge
or use laxatives.

The causes of night eating are not well understood, but it appears
to involve a disturbance of the body's internal clock. Even though the
normal sleep/wake cycle is intact, appetite is clearly highest at night.
It seems to be triggered by stress or depression, but there may be a
genetic predisposition. There is even a suggestion that the pituitary
gland in the brain is malfunctioning, causing defective secretion of
stress hormones such as cortisol. Some researchers suggest that sufferers are self-medicating with food, unconsciously aware that carbohydrates stimulate "feel-good" chemicals such as serotonin.

What can you do about it?

If you think you have night eating syndrome, it's important that you
contact your doctor and ask for a full physical examination and a
referral to an eating disorder specialist. There are medications that
can help reset the body's natural circadian (daily) rhythm and lift feelings of depression. Optimal treatment for night eating syndrome is
still being developed, but a dietitian can help with healthy, low-GI
meal plans that will leave you less vulnerable to the nighttime
munchies.

What You Need to Do—
Activity and Exercise

*O*nce you have been through a weight-loss phase, exercise and activity become more important than ever. The single most important difference between long-term weight losers and weight gainers is the amount of physical activity they build into their day. Quite simply, exercise has to be your first priority. At the end of your 12-week Action Plan, you should be fitter and capable of doing more than you were able to at the start. The aim in the Doing It for Life phase is to maintain the same activity level of Week 12 (see pages 160–63), but build in different forms of exercise so that you don't become bored. Setting new goals and enjoying what you do are both critical.

■

FOOD MINUS EXERCISE EQUALS FAT!

■

To appreciate the importance of exercise and activity, let's take a look at the big picture. It is not how much fat or energy is used during a single bout of activity, but how it all adds up over the months and years that matters. The fact is that most of us gain weight very slowly over the years—on average gaining 1 to 2 pounds every year. So ten years down the road, you weigh 11 to 22 pounds more. Similarly, small amounts of activity may seem unimportant in the short term— you can't detect a change on the scales—but they add up over the long term. In the table below, consider how many pounds of fat you potentially "save" if you take five minutes here and five minutes there to be active. Every little bit counts!

Take five minutes every day to:	Potential saving in pounds of fat*	
	in 1 year	in 5 years
Take the stairs instead of the elevator	8	40
Weed one patch of the garden	1	7
Rake the lawn	1	7
Vacuum the living room	1	8
Walk 500 feet from the car to the office	1	8
Carry the groceries 500 feet back to the car	2	10

*Figures are based on a 154-pound person.

This shows us that all those seemingly small actions where we *choose* to take the more active option really do add up in the long run. It won't hurt you to park your car at the farthest end of the parking lot. It might not feel as if climbing one flight of stairs makes a difference. But it does—you can save yourself 2 or 4 pounds of fat over the course of a year. Similarly, even if you have just five minutes rather than thirty minutes to fit in some exercise, do it anyway. It is abundantly clear why active people find it much easier to avoid regaining weight.

Keep an activity journal for a week and record any exercise you do in addition to active choices you have made. Review it at the end of the week and see how well you have done and whether you are being as active as you can be. See the example journals below.

Karen's journal

Monday: Walked the dog (30 minutes), used the stairs instead of the escalator in the shopping center, and walked 5 minutes to the local store for more milk instead of taking the car.

Tuesday: Raining so didn't walk the dog. Spent most of the day at my desk—only activity was a short walk to the café for lunch.

Wednesday: Attended a yoga class.

Thursday: Walked the dog (30 minutes), spring-cleaned the house for the whole afternoon—exhausted, but feel a great sense of achievement.

Friday: Went to an indoor cycling class at my local health club—loved it! Much better than sitting on a bike in the gym on my own. Felt so good I walked home afterward—20 minutes.

Saturday: Took the dog for a long walk (60 minutes) first thing this morning. Went shopping for the afternoon—on my feet for 4 hours. Carried my shopping home (a 15-minute walk) instead of taking the bus.

Sunday: Lazy day at home and didn't do much activity other than press the buttons on the television remote!

Review:

Karen had a fairly good week activity-wise. She accumulated 160 minutes of walking, not counting all the walking of an afternoon's shopping, as well as a yoga class, an indoor cycling class, and the extra energy expended in taking the stairs, cleaning the house, and carrying shopping bags. Looking back at her week, however, Karen realizes there were two days when she did almost no activity or exercise.

She enjoyed her fitness class so much that she has decided to add a second class on a Tuesday night to ensure she is active for six days of the week, and she has chosen to keep Sunday as her day of rest and recuperation.

Tom's journal

Monday–Friday: Left the car at home and walked to the train station (10 minutes), which meant a short 5-minute walk to the office at the other end. At lunchtime, instead of eating at my desk, I bought a sandwich and walked to the nearby park (5 minutes there and 5 minutes back) and enjoyed a 20-minute break—the fresh air and break from my desk actually helped to keep me focused for the afternoon, whereas I usually have an "energy slump" after lunch.

Adding in the walk to and from the train station each day, I have accumulated 40 minutes of walking into my day! I'm amazed at how much better I feel without adding exercise time commitments to my day.

Saturday: Took the kids to the park in the afternoon armed with a Frisbee and a football—comfortably spent an hour having fun, and the kids loved it, too.

Sunday: Washed and vacuumed the car by hand with a little help from the kids (enticed with some extra pocket money). It took us only half an hour, but the car looks great and saved me some money on the usual car wash charge (despite having to bribe the kids).

Review:

Tom works in an office and, although he played sports and was much more active when he was younger, he has found it increasingly difficult to find the time for exercise while working long hours and spending time with his young family. Tom had decided to try to fit in an accumulated thirty minutes of activity into his day—let's take a look at how he achieved this. He actually built forty minutes of accumulated activity into his day by walking to the train station instead of taking his car and going for a short stroll at lunchtime. Adding to this the extra activities with the kids on the weekend, Tom has drastically increased his weekly activity.

In the bottle before you is a pill, a marvel of modern medicine that will regulate gene transcription throughout your body, help prevent heart disease, stroke, diabetes, obesity, and 12 kinds of cancer—plus gallstones and diverticulitis (inflammation of the intestines). Expect the pill to improve your strength and balance as well as your blood lipid profile. Your bones will become stronger. You'll grow new capillaries in your heart, your skeletal muscles and your brain, improving blood flow and the delivery of oxygen and nutrients. Your attention span will increase. If you have arthritis, your symptoms will improve. The pill will help you regulate your appetite and you'll probably find you prefer healthier foods. You'll feel better, younger even, and you will test younger according to a variety of physiologic measures. Your blood volume will increase and you will burn fats better. Even your immune system will be stimulated. There is just one catch.

There's no such pill. The prescription is exercise.

Jonathan Shaw, *Harvard Magazine* (March–April 2004)

In short, building exercise into your life is vital. There really couldn't be a more powerful means of improving your health while looking and feeling better. There is much controversy in scientific research regarding nutrition, but there is unanimity over the benefits of exercise.

This does not mean you need to go and join a gym or start pounding the streets every night. There are lots of options, and finding what sort of exercise is suitable and enjoyable to you is the key to success. Use the exercise selector on pages 205–210 to help you figure out which form of exercise will work best for you.

TYPES OF EXERCISE

While exercise works through three different systems, as illustrated below, many forms of exercise work more than one system—and sometimes all three. Cycling, for example, is primarily an aerobic exercise, but also involves resistance training for the legs, as they have to push against a force. Yoga is usually thought of as primarily improving flexibility, yet holding the poses involves a good deal of resistance training, using your body weight as resistance.

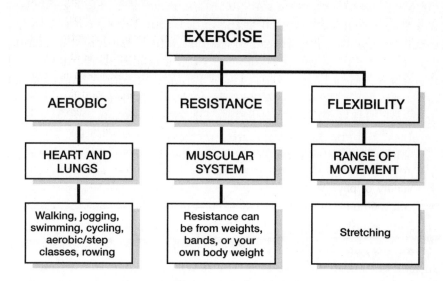

In your initial 12-week Action Plan, we focused on aerobic exercise (walking) and resistance training in the form of key exercises you could do at home. Both of these forms of exercise are most effective in helping you to lose body fat, and they continue to be important from now on in helping you to avoid regaining weight. This doesn't mean that flexibility training is any less important—you should always stretch at the end of your exercise session—but spending more time on the types of exercise that will specifically help your weight control is just good time management. Let's take a look at some popular forms of exercise and see where they fit in with this model.

Walking and jogging

We chose walking as the suggested form of exercise in the 12-week Action Plan for good reason—it's undoubtedly one of the best forms of exercise you can do for your health, and almost anyone can do it. Continuing with your walking program may be all you want to do at this point, and that is fine.

If, however, you are ready to step up your fitness a little more, you can raise the intensity, building up to a jog, or increase the time you spend walking.

Aerobics classes

As the name suggests, these are primarily aerobic workouts, although many will also incorporate some resistance exercises, and a good class will always include a stretch at the end. Group fitness classes are an excellent way to motivate you to exercise a little harder—the combination of uplifting music, guidance from a qualified instructor, and the group atmosphere makes classes fun and effective. Don't be put off by the old "leg warmers and thong leotards" image! Times have changed, and there are now classes to suit everyone—choose from aerobics, step, boxing, martial arts, or circuit training. Classes are run in health clubs, recreational centers, universities, and local schools all around the country.

Cycling

If you love to get outdoors and to exercise alone, then cycling may be for you. Cycling is primarily aerobic exercise, but it also involves some resistance training for the legs. The downside is that you will need to invest in a decent bike and helmet—cycling shorts and shoes are also a good idea. Once you are geared up and ready to go, this is an excellent form of exercise to keep burning the calories. Of course, biking needn't be a solo activity—try getting the whole family involved on the weekend, or join a cycling group in your area for organized routes and social contact. The other option is to go to an indoor group cycling class at your local health club. These are led by instructors, with motivating music to inspire you to give your best.

Rowing and kayaking

A good option if you live near the water and like to be outdoors. Rowing and kayaking mainly provide aerobic exercise, but since you are also using both upper- and lower-body strength, you incorporate a good deal of resistance training at the same time.

Tennis, squash, and other racket sports

These sports provide effective aerobic exercise; plus, the social aspect helps you to keep it up. If you have never played before, book yourself in for a program of lessons—then you'll meet fellow beginners to play with on a regular basis.

Golf
While not as intense as some of the other forms of exercise, golf does take a long time to play, and can be a great way to assist your weight loss. Of course, you need to walk to gain the benefits, so leave the golf cart at the clubhouse!

Weight training
The people who really need to weight train are not the young guns who can be spotted pumping iron at your local gym, but the rest of us. As you already know, increasing your muscle mass raises your metabolic rate and helps you burn more fat all of the time, but did you know that weight training also strengthens your bones and can help prevent weight gain as we age? This means that weight training is important for women approaching menopause, those at risk of osteoporosis, seniors, and anyone who wants to control their weight. Health clubs now have sophisticated equipment that ensures that you train effectively and safely—or you can work with resistance bands or join a weights-based group exercise class.

Team sports
If you enjoy the competition and camaraderie of team sports, then find a local team playing the sport you like. You could try soccer, volleyball, hockey, basketball, rugby, or baseball. All of these offer great aerobic training, and clubs often have a program that also incorporates resistance and flexibility training.

Pilates and yoga
These classes focus more on flexibility, but also have a good element of resistance training—as you will know if you have ever tried to hold a yoga pose or taken part in a Pilates class. They have very little aerobic benefit, however, and, while they are a good addition to your exercise program, ensure that you also include some form of aerobic training. That said, there are different forms of both classes—for example, Ashtanga yoga is far more energetic and demanding than other more relaxing and meditative forms of yoga.

Swimming

Water provides fifteen times more resistance than air. For this reason, working out in water can be extremely effective. If you are very over-weight or suffer from arthritis or an injury, getting into the water offers a safe and effective means of exercising. The water supports your body weight, your muscles work against the resistance of the water, and you won't feel sore afterward (muscle soreness comes mainly from muscles lengthening under resistance—in water, the opposing muscle takes over, so muscles only ever have to contract against the resistance). You can choose from swimming laps or joining an aqua aerobics class in which an instructor will lead you through a series of exercises in the water.

Dancing

Dance classes are a fabulous way to get active. Not only are they lots of fun, but many are also a great way to meet new friends and social-ize. Any kind of dancing is suitable—choose from jazz, salsa, Scottish dancing, line dancing, ballet, and ballroom—the choices are endless. See what appeals to you and what is available in your area. The adver-tisements in the back of your local newspaper are a good starting point.

■

WHATEVER TYPE OF EXERCISE YOU DECIDE ON, THE TWO IMPORTANT FACTORS ARE THAT YOU ENJOY THE EXERCISE AND THAT YOU DO IT REGULARLY.

■

THE EXERCISE SELECTOR

The key to making exercise a regular part of your life is to find something that you enjoy and look forward to. That's not to say that there won't be times when you have to motivate yourself to get to your exercise session, but finding the motivation will be infinitely easier if you are then rewarded by a fun, enjoyable session that leaves you invigorated. If you hate running and are not an early-morning person, then choosing to get up for a 6 AM run before work will not last beyond the first couple of weeks. Similarly, if you live in a rural area, more than thirty minutes' drive from the nearest fitness center, then attending a group fitness class will become difficult to maintain in the long run. Use the following questionnaire to help you to identify what form of exercise might suit you best.

- ◗ For each question, highlight the answer row that applies to you with a fluorescent pen.
- ◗ Then, for each activity column, add up your scores and enter the total at the bottom.
- ◗ This is your total score for each activity.

	Walking/ jogging	Aerobics	Cycling	Kayaking
Personal Details				
Age				
Under 35	0	0	0	0
35-49	0	0	0	0
50-59	2	3	3	1
60+	✓ 4	7	7	2
Body frame				
Small/medium	0	0	0	0
Large	3	2	0	0

Exercise Questionnaire

	Walking/ jogging	Aerobics	Cycling	Kayaking
Are you more than a little overweight?				
No	0	0	0	0
Yes	4	4	3	3
Are you an indoor or outdoor person?				
Indoor	7	0	6	8
Outdoor	0	1	1	0
Are you self-conscious about exercising in pulic?				
No	0	0	0	0
Yes	5	8	4	0
How competitive are you?				
Highly	3	1	5	3
Moderately	0	1	4	3
Not very	0	0	2	0
Are you prepared to pay more than $30 a week to exercise?				
Yes	0	0	0	0
No	0	8	2	0
Are you suffering limiting injuries to any of the following:				
Legs/ankles/knees?	9	9	4	0
Shoulders/arms?	1	7	2	7
Hip?	9	9	3	1
Back?	5	10	5	5

Weight training	Ball games	Yoga/ Pilates	Swimming	Dancing	Circuit training	Skipping/ stepping
0	0	0	0	0	0	0
0	4	0	0	1	0	3
1	5	0	0	3	1	5
9	6	0	0	4	✓4	8
0	0	0	0	0	0	0
0	2	2	0	2	2	4
0	0	0	0	0	0	0
0	6	4	0	4	✓3	5
0	0	0	0	0	0	0
1	0	4	2	0	1	5
0	0	0	0	0	0	0
3	5	3	4	7	0	0
1	0	8	3	8	2	8
0	2	4	3	5	✓1	5
0	8	0	3	0	0	0
0	0	0	0	0	0	0
8	4	4	1	4	0	0
1	7	3	1	7	5	9
6	5	4	3	2	4	4
1	7	6	3	7	3	8
2	6	3	2	6	4	5

	Walking/ jogging	Aerobics	Cycling	Kayaking

Exercise Questionnaire

Are you NOT within easy reach (say 15 minutes) of any of the following:

	Walking/ jogging	Aerobics	Cycling	Kayaking
Pool/lake/sea?	0	0	0	10
Park/open space?	5	0	0	0
Fitness center?	0	5	0	0
Sports facilities?	0	0	0	0
Safe bike routes?	0	0	10	0

How much time can you give 3-4 days a week for exercise?

<20 mins	4	9	3	6
20-40 mins	0	2	0	2
>40 mins	0	0	0	0

How do you prefer to exercise?

Alone	0	0	0	0
With a friend	1	9	3	1
In a group	2	0	6	3

Total Test Score

Calculate your **interest score** for each activity

- If you think you would definitely enjoy carrying out the activity regularly, give yourself an interest score of 100.
- If you think you may enjoy carrying out the activity regularly, give yourself an interest score of 90.
- If the activity doesn't appeal to you, give yourself an interest score of 80.

Insert your interest score for each activity into the corresponding space.

Weight training	Ball games	Yoga/ Pilates	Swimming	Dancing	Circuit training	Skipping/ stepping
0	0	0	10	0	0	0
0	0	0	0	0	0	0
9	4	5	0	3	0	0
0	10	0	0	0	0	0
0	0	0	0	0	0	0
5	10	5	10	10	3	3
0	4	0	4	2	0	0
0	0	0	0	0	0	0
0	10	3	0	5	1	0
0	0	4	2	0	1	3
8	0	0	2	0	✓1	6

	Walking/Jogging	Aerobics	Cycling	Kayaking	Weight training	Ball games	Yoga/Pilates	Swimming	Dancing	Circuit training	Skipping/stepping
Interest Score										8	

Calculate a **final score** for each activity by subtracting the **total test score** from the **interest score** for each activity.

	Walking/Jogging	Aerobics	Cycling	Kayaking	Weight training	Ball games	Yoga/Pilates	Swimming	Dancing	Circuit training	Skipping/stepping
Final score (Interest Score *minus* total test score)											

The activity with the highest final score will generally be the most appropriate form of exercise for you. If there are several activities at the top falling within about 5 points of each other, choose the one you think you would prefer, or combine them for a varied program. It's a good idea to combine at least a couple of activities to maintain your interest in your program and challenge your body in different ways.

USING A PEDOMETER

A pedometer is a nifty little tool that is highly effective in helping you achieve a walking goal. Inexpensive and available at good sports shops and department stores, it looks a bit like a pager that you clip to your waistband or belt in the morning. It counts the number of steps you take during the day, which can be a real eye-opener as to how active you really are—you may well be completely shocked at how few steps you actually take during a normal day!

There are now guidelines to advise us on how many steps we should be aiming for, and these are shown below. You may have to build yourself up to these levels slowly. Wear your pedometer for the first week of Doing It for Life, and at the end of each day, record the number of steps you took. Work out your average daily steps at the end of the week and add 30 percent. This is your new goal for the next two to three weeks. Once you are achieving the new step goal easily, add a further 30 percent. Repeat this process, taking as long as you need at each stage, until you are meeting the goals below.

- For optimum health: aim to achieve 7,500 steps per day.
- For weight loss during the 12-week Action Plan: aim to achieve 10,000 steps per day.
- To avoid regaining weight: aim to achieve 12,500 steps per day.

Of course, the pedometer only counts the actual walking that you do, and not other activities. The following table gives you an idea of how many steps are equivalent to fifteen minutes of certain activities. Using these guidelines, you can reduce your daily step goal on days when you engage in some other exercise or activity.

15 minutes of activity	Equivalent number of steps
Moderate sexual activity	500
Standing while watering lawn or garden	600
Vigorous sexual activity	750
Clearing and washing dishes	900
Standing while cooking at the barbecue	950
Standing while playing with kids	1,100
Carpentry—general workshop	1,200
Playing Frisbee	1,200
Bowling	1,200
Playing golf at the driving range	1,200
Food shopping with a cart	1,400
General house cleaning	1,400
Bicycling moderately (11 mph)	1,600
Raking the lawn	1,600
Playing actively with kids	1,600
Sweeping	1,600
Paddleboat peddling	1,600
Horseback riding	1,600
Playing table tennis	1,600
Washing the car by hand	1,850
Spreading soil with a shovel	1,950
Cleaning gutters of house	2,000
Walking/running while playing vigorously with kids	2,000
Digging or cultivating the garden	2,000
Mowing the lawn with a hand mower	2,350
Moving furniture	2,350
Carrying bricks	3,150
Using heavy tools—e.g., shovel or crow bar	3,150

WHAT ABOUT JOINING A HEALTH CLUB?

Health clubs are a great way to build exercise into your life—you have expert advice from qualified instructors, group fitness classes to choose from, and a program designed for you in the gym; many also have a pool, squash courts, or an associated running club.

Nevertheless, your first visit can be a little daunting. Do your research first and find a club that meets your needs:

- Is it within a 15-minute drive of either your home or work?
- If you have young children, is there a babysitting service?
- What are the opening hours—if you want to go in the early morning or late evening, are there classes at these times?
- If you think you would enjoy swimming or aqua classes, is there a pool?
- Will an instructor provide a gym program to get you started?
- What are the membership fee options and what is the termination clause if you wish to end your membership?

WHAT ABOUT A PERSONAL TRAINER?

There is no doubt that employing a personal trainer is a terrific way to improve your fitness and progress toward your goals. A good trainer will provide an individualized, progressive program as well as much-needed motivation and support. Many personal trainers now provide services for a reasonable rate, and you can choose to use a health club or train outdoors. A good way to bring the cost down is to train with a small group of three or four others with similar fitness levels. For more information on personal trainers, see page 217.

What if I don't have access to a personal trainer or health club, or can't afford it?

Use the "buddy system"—you can get all the support and motivation you need from exercising with a buddy who has similar goals. Having an appointment to go walking or swimming with a friend makes it harder to be distracted or find an excuse to put it off. Remember, you are also offering the same motivation and support to your buddy, so that you are both more likely to succeed.

SETTING AN EXAMPLE FOR THE KIDS

We know we can't force kids to exercise, but you can lead by example. If they see you lounging on the sofa every night, eating chips and watching television for hours, then, inevitably, they copy that behavior. Kids of active parents or guardians are far more likely to be active themselves—if not now, then in the future. You may even persuade them to come exercising with you—stranger things have happened!

Get the kids moving, too
1. Restrict periods of extended inactivity such as watching television or videos or playing computer games.
2. Invent projects to create at home (like a go-cart or a bird feeder).
3. Don't encourage sedentary behavior over activity. (You may have to delete "sit down and be quiet" from your vocabulary.)
4. Make sure the kids aren't watching *you* watching television.
5. Let them see you being active.
6. Don't chauffeur them everywhere; let them use public transportation.
7. Don't confine them to the four walls of home or school.
8. Don't restrict spontaneous decisions to be active.
9. Put the ride-on toys and trampoline where they catch attention.
10. Prepare food with their help; for example, they could help you with a special dish.

Practical ways to reduce television watching
1. Make a rule and enforce it: no more than 12 hours per week.
2. Schedule the programs you will watch for the week.
3. Rearrange the furniture so there is more room for movement.
4. Do stretches and floor exercises while you watch.
5. Put the television in a naturally light room to discourage daytime viewing.
6. Turn on the stereo instead.
7. Play now—do homework later. (The kids will love this!)
8. During the commercial breaks, try to get a small chore done.
9. Anything is better than nothing.
10. Combine television watching with the ironing (it's not just Mom's job, either).

HOW MUCH DO YOU NEED TO DO?

Now that you have decided what types of exercise you would enjoy and are going to suit you, plan how they will fit into your week. If you write exactly what you are going to do in your journal and treat it like any other appointment, you will ensure that you stick to the plan.

Try to do something active on most days, and add the following:

▶ Three cardiovascular sessions—this could be a group fitness class, cycling, a brisk walk, or swimming.

▶ Two resistance workouts—either continue with your program from Week 12 of the Action Plan or join a weights-based group fitness class, or have a program designed for you at your local health club. Yoga and Pilates classes will also improve your strength and muscle tone, though to a lesser extent.

What Else You Can Do—The Last Tools in the Toolbox

FIND A GOOD DIETITIAN

*D*ietitians **have professionally** recognized qualifications in human nutrition. They can provide specific advice tailored to your current eating habits and food preferences, and will work with you to set realistic and achievable goals. They will help you understand the relationship between food and health and guide you in making dietary choices that optimize your lifestyle. Dietitians practice as individual professionals and are available through most public hospitals and in private practice. To find a dietitian, look in the Yellow Pages under Dietitians or call the American Dietetic Association's Consumer Nutrition Hotline (800-366-1655); or go to the ADA's home page: www.eatright.org. Make sure that the person you choose has the letters "RD" (Registered Dietitian) after his or her name.

> ### What to expect when you see a dietitian
>
> Your first visit to a dietitian will generally take about an hour and will begin with the collection of personal details, such as your weight and medical history, usual eating patterns and activity levels, and goals and expectations. This information helps the dietitian to assess your needs and provide information and education relevant to you.

FIND A GOOD PERSONAL TRAINER

If you belong to a health club, you should be able to find a personal trainer there. For working out in your own home or outdoors, look in your local newspaper or search online for someone in your area. Ask to see their qualifications—they should be certified in training. Any good trainer will offer you at least one complimentary session to "try before you buy"—to make sure you like the style of your trainer and can work well with him or her before you sign up for a number of sessions.

■

TWENTY MINUTES OF EXERCISE GIVES YOU A MOOD BOOST AND A NATURAL HIGH.

■

> ### What to expect when you see a personal trainer
>
> In your first session, a good personal trainer will quiz you on your current lifestyle, your goals, and what you expect from working with him or her. He or she will then work out a program to best guide you toward reaching those goals.
>
> Discuss payment options with the trainer during your first session. You should expect to have at least the first session free of charge to see if you are a compatible team. If you are not sure, try out another trainer.

WHAT YOU NEED TO KNOW ABOUT USING DRUGS TO TREAT WEIGHT CONCERNS

If you have tried the Action Plan and followed it up with the Doing It for Life phase and have seen no reduction in your weight, you might want to think about discussing drug treatments with your doctor.

First of all, you should be aware that your doctor won't even consider prescribing any drug therapy until you have actively pursued a dietary and physical activity change for at least three months. If at the end of that period you have lost little weight (say, less than 5 percent of your initial weight), then drug therapy *might* be an option. Your doctor will consider the risks against the benefits in your individual case. Even when drug therapy is initiated, however, it's never used as sole therapy, but as an adjunct to a diet and exercise program.

Drugs for the treatment of obesity have gotten a bad reputation and many doctors are reluctant to use them. This is unfortunate, because appropriate drug treatment can be life-saving. In the past, drugs were used inappropriately, regaining weight was common, and some drugs were associated with addiction and serious side effects. Nowadays, most of these drugs have been withdrawn from use. Those that are used today have been subjected to large international clinical trials and are safer than the drugs prescribed ten or twenty years ago.

There are two principal drugs currently available throughout much of the world, including the United States, Australia, New Zealand, and the UK, for the management of obesity. The first is called *orlistat*. It is a lipase inhibitor, a substance that blocks the digestion of fat (lipids). In practice, 10 to 30 percent of fat eaten is not absorbed and is excreted in the feces. Over the course of six to twelve months, orlistat has been shown to produce a 10 percent weight loss, compared to only a 6 percent weight loss in patients who took the placebo. This might not seem to be a big difference, but it can make a huge difference to blood-glucose and blood-lipid levels and therefore reduce the risk of developing diabetes and cardiovascular disease. During treatment with orlistat, it's absolutely essential to eat a low-fat diet to reduce the severity of the gastrointestinal side effects. These include flatulence with discharge, oily evacuation, and fecal incontinence. Not to be taken lightly! Fortunately, the side effects lessen with time, and most people stick to the treatment. A general vitamin supplement should be taken alongside orlistat, because fat-soluble vitamins can be mal-absorbed along with the fat.

The second drug commonly prescribed for treating overweight people is *sibutramine*. It's an appetite suppressant, acting on the nerve pathways in the brain to inhibit food intake. It has been subjected to widespread international trials and is safe for use in uncomplicated obesity. It should not be prescribed to people with any form of heart disease or who have had a stroke. It can also interfere with the metabolism of other drugs, such as antidepressants and blood pressure medication, so caution is important.

In the past, caffeine and ephedrine have also been used in pharmacological amounts to rev up metabolism and increase energy expenditure. In excess, however, there are serious side effects, and these substances are *not* currently recommended for the treatment of obesity. Natural ways to rev up your metabolism are better—get moving and avoid skipping meals.

What about the magic bullets of the future? Scientists are carrying out trials with hormones that control appetite such as leptin and cholecystokinin (CCK). Substances that block appetite receptors in the brain are also under investigation. But don't get too excited—blocking one route simply means other pathways come into play. Our bodies have evolved a myriad of ways to ensure we eat up, even when we feel otherwise inclined.

If you have done your best with a serious attempt at weight loss over three months, even with the additional help of a dietitian or personal trainer, and still feel dissatisfied with the amount of weight loss, we recommend a visit to your doctor. If you are markedly overweight—if your waist circumference is over 40 inches (male) or 35 inches (female)—he or she might refer you to an endocrinologist who specializes in obesity management. Apart from medication, there are surgical interventions to help those who are extremely overweight.

HOW ABOUT ALTERNATIVE TREATMENTS?

Alternative treatments have become increasingly popular in all areas of health and well-being. Walk into any health food store and you are faced with a plethora of supplements all claiming to help you lose weight. The advertising and marketing of these products are powerfully persuasive—often using before and after photos of people who have reportedly transformed their bodies entirely just by using the advertised product. Is there any truth behind these claims?

The short answer is, unfortunately, no. If there were an easy answer to weight loss, then so many of us wouldn't be struggling! One reason supplements may seem to work in the short term is the so-called placebo effect—if you believe strongly enough that something will help you to lose weight, it probably will—not because the supplement is achieving what it claims, but because with this perceived helping hand you manage to reduce your energy intake, at least for a short while.

Nevertheless, there are a small number of products that do plausibly aid weight loss and show promise for the future, although even these few will never provide the miracle cure. At best, they may be useful as an adjunct treatment to the type of lifestyle modifications we have laid out in this book—these will always be the cornerstone of achieving better health and, in the process, successful weight control.

One problem with supplements is that if they are successful in assisting weight loss, then inevitably there will be side effects. This is true whether the supplement is a drug or a "natural" product. Don't be fooled by the word "natural"—this does not necessarily mean "safe." In fact, many herbal products can be extremely dangerous, because there is little control over how much of the active ingredient is present—unlike drugs, which are strictly regulated to provide a standardized dose. This can mean you either don't get enough of the active ingredient to make a difference, or you get too much, increasing the risk of unpleasant side effects.

Many over-the-counter weight-loss products contain different combinations of the same ingredients. These include the following:

Ma Huang (ephedra)

Ma Huang is the Chinese name for the plant ephedra. The active ingredient is ephedrine, and in Europe supplements containing ephedrine and caffeine combinations have been popular for weight loss. In the United States and Australia, however, Ma Huang and ephedrine have been banned due to their serious side effects, including elevated blood pressure and heart rate, insomnia, agitation, dry mouth, gastrointestinal upsets, and, in some cases, death. In light of these safety concerns, it's prudent to avoid the supplement.

Herbs reported to reduce appetite and/or raise metabolic rate

These include brindleberry, gymnema, bladder wrack, dandelion, calendula, blue flag, ginseng, kelp, and garcinia cambogia. None of these extracts have been conclusively shown to be effective. One possible exception is a fruit acid extracted from the rind of brindleberry, called HCA (hydroxycitric acid), which may enhance weight loss when combined with a low-energy diet. A more recent, more rigorous study, however, found no such effect.

Fiber—often as guar gum or psyllium

Since fiber absorbs water in the gut and swells, it can help you to feel full after a meal. There is little evidence, however, that taking fiber in supplement form will help you to lose weight. You will find it best to stick with a high-fiber, low-GI diet that has proven health benefits.

Chitosan

Chitosan comes from the shells of crustaceans and has been shown to bind fat. The theory is that it can therefore bind fat in your gut, preventing absorption. Unfortunately, this does not seem to happen in real life, and these claims remain unsubstantiated.

Chromium picolinate

We need small amounts of the mineral chromium for correct carbohydrate and fat metabolism, and, in particular, for making sure that insulin works effectively. In a rather giant leap, it was therefore suggested that taking chromium in supplement form would reduce insulin resistance and encourage fat burning while preserving lean muscle. A small amount of evidence does show an improvement in insulin action in people with type 2 diabetes, but the majority of studies have shown no effect. The picolinate form found in most supplements has been shown to damage DNA in rats, and while it is not known if this occurs in humans, we should at least exercise caution until further research is carried out.

Carnitine and choline

These supplements claim to assist in fat mobilization. While they are involved in fat transport within the body, there is no evidence that taking them in supplement form can help you to lose body fat.

Furthermore, these substances are found naturally in meat and dairy foods and so can be consumed easily in your normal diet.

Capsaicin

This is the chemical responsible for the spicy bite to chili peppers and cayenne powder. There is some evidence that capsaicin can boost your metabolic rate, and this research led to a short craze in the UK of eating hot curries in an attempt to lose weight! While the effect can be measured when consumed in supplement form, the increase is so minor as to have no promising effect on weight loss.

To summarize, none of the currently available supplements have proven efficacy and safety, and in buying them you are more likely to lighten your wallet than lighten your weight on the scales. Even those that hold some promise can help only as part of a total lifestyle-modification program. Our advice is to save your money and put all of your energies into changing the factors that we know will count in the long run—what you eat and how often you move!

LOOKING FORWARD TO
THE ONE-YEAR MARK

A year of following the Low GI Diet Revolution will give you a new lease on life. Having lost at least 5 to 10 percent of your initial body weight, you will be fitting into clothes one or two sizes smaller, you will look and feel terrific, and you will feel an undeniable buzz every time you have done your exercise for the day. Most importantly, you will have kept off the weight you lost and developed the confidence and know-how that ensure you keep it off for the rest of your life. Sure, there will be times when you regain a little, but that's normal and it shouldn't faze you, as you know you can repeat the Action Plan and shed the pounds at any stage. You will have learned exactly what it takes to keep your weight under control through the recommendations in this chapter. It is not just about eating, but also about physical activity and balancing the energy equation. You have adopted a lifestyle, not a "diet."

The amount of weight you have lost may not take you back to your weight at age 18 or 25, but it doesn't matter. The weight you lose in this first year is what makes the world of difference to your health and well-being. While it might not be at the forefront of your mind right now, living the healthy low-GI life will be giving you lots of value-added benefits, such as reducing the likelihood that you will develop diabetes, heart disease, arthritis, cancer, and a number of other diseases. Your quality of life will remain high as the years advance, and you will be in the best shape possible to meet the challenges and pleasures of middle and older age. Putting your health first gives you the best possible chance of achieving not only lifelong dreams, but everything else life puts on your plate.

■

READ THE LANGUAGE OF YOUR BODY— NOTICE WHEN YOU FEEL MOST ALIVE AND DO MORE OF THAT.

■

PART FOUR

Recipes

Nutritional Information

The following recipes are quick, delicious, low-GI, and super-easy to make. They are full of healthy ingredients, such as whole grains, lean meats, fish and seafood, legumes, and fresh fruits and vegetables. The recipes reflect the philosophy of the Low GI Diet Revolution and emphasize:

- Low-GI carbs
- Monounsaturated and omega-3 fats
- A moderate to high level of protein

All the recipes in this section have been analyzed using a computerized nutrient-analysis program, and the energy, protein, carbohydrate, fat, and fiber content per serving are shown. If the recipe is rich in particular micronutrients, we have identified them for you.

GI rating

Low GI = 55 or less
Moderate GI = 56–69
High GI = 70 or more

GL rating

Low = 10 or less
Moderate = 11–19
High = 20 or more

Where the recipe has a high GL, we suggest serving it with foods that have little glycemic impact, such as salads, vegetables, and lean meat or seafood.

In the recipes where eggs are used, we recommend omega-3-enriched eggs. Where honey is used, we recommend using pure floral honey, which has a lower GI.

So, that's the nutrition part of it. Now it's time to start cooking and embark on your low-GI journey to fitness and good health. Enjoy!

Light Meals and Brunches

BREAKFAST ON THE GO

A quick and healthy breakfast drink.

PREPARATION TIME 5 minutes ■ **COOKING TIME** none ■ **SERVES** 2

PER SERVING:

Calories 353

Protein 27 g

Fat 4 g (saturated 1 g)

Carbohydrate 55 g

Fiber 3 g

GI Low

GL Moderate

1 Combine the ingredients in a blender.

2 Process until smooth and frothy.

3 Pour into two glasses, drink, and go!

2 cups low-fat milk or soy beverage

½ cup low-fat plain yogurt

1 cup strawberries, hulled and chopped (optional)

1 large, ripe banana, roughly chopped

1 egg (optional)

1 tablespoon pure honey

1 tablespoon All-Bran or wheat germ

EGG AND BACON TARTS

These tarts are delicious, simple, and healthy to make for a breakfast or brunch. The high fat content makes them a great weekend treat.

PREPARATION TIME 10 minutes ■ **COOKING TIME** 20–25 minutes ■ **SERVES** 2

PER SERVING:

Calories 386

Protein 28 g

Fat 18 g (saturated 6 g)

Carbohydrate 30 g

Fiber 4 g

GI Low

GL Low

4 slices whole-grain bread

Spray olive oil or canola oil

4 small eggs

2 slices bacon, trimmed and finely chopped

¼ cup reduced-fat cheese, grated

1 tablespoon parsley, chopped

1 Preheat the oven to 350°F.

2 Trim any thick or hard crusts from the bread and flatten each slice by rolling gently with a rolling pin.

3 Spray a medium-cup muffin pan with the oil and gently push each slice of bread into its own cup to line it. Spray again.

4 Break an egg into each cup—don't worry if it overflows a little. Top each with some bacon, cheese, and parsley.

5 Bake for 20 to 25 minutes or until set.

VEGETABLE FRITTATA

A lovely light lunch, this frittata is also great for picnics. It's a good source of folic acid and rich in beta-carotene. Serve fresh sour-dough bread alongside.

PREPARATION TIME 20 minutes ■ **COOKING TIME** 45 minutes ■ Makes 4 wedges

PER SERVING:

Calories 190

Protein 12 g

Fat 9 g (saturated 3 g)

Carbohydrate 14 g

Fiber 4 g

GI Low

GL Low

1 teaspoon olive oil

1 small onion, finely chopped

1 clove garlic, crushed

2 cups sweet potato, grated

2 small zucchini, grated

¼ cup basil leaves, finely
  chopped

⅓ cup reduced-fat cheese,
  grated

salt and freshly ground black
  pepper, to taste

4 eggs, lightly beaten

6 cherry tomatoes, halved

To serve

6 cups mixed salad greens

squeeze of lemon juice

1 Preheat the oven to 350°F. Lightly grease an 8-inch round cake pan and line the base with nonstick parchment paper.

2 Heat the olive oil in a nonstick frying pan and cook the onion and garlic for 4 minutes, or until soft. Add the sweet potato and zucchini and cook, stirring, for 3 minutes or until softened slightly.

3 Transfer the vegetable mixture to a bowl and cool slightly. Mix in the basil and cheese, and season with salt and pepper. Stir to combine evenly. Fold in the eggs, and pour the mixture into the prepared pan. Smooth the surface.

4 Arrange the cherry tomatoes over the mixture, cut side up, and press in gently. Bake for 45 minutes, until set and golden. Leave in the pan until just cool enough to handle, then turn out and quickly invert right-side-up onto a plate.

5 Cut the frittata into wedges and serve with salad greens, lightly dressed with lemon juice.

SALMON AND DILL OMELET WITH TOMATO SALAD

*T*his omelet is a fantastic source of omega-3 fats, thanks to the salmon and eggs. Serve with salad and rye bread.

PREPARATION TIME 15 minutes ■ **COOKING TIME** 5 minutes ■ **SERVES** 2

PER SERVING:
(with bread and salad):
Calories 767
Protein 42 g
Fat 45 g (saturated 12 g)
Carbohydrate 47 g
Fiber 10 g
GI Low
GL High

4 eggs, at room temperature
2 tablespoons low-fat milk
1 tablespoon fresh dill, chopped
salt and freshly ground black
    pepper, to taste
2 teaspoons canola margarine
1 cup baby spinach leaves
¼ pound smoked salmon, cut
    into thin strips
¼ cup Parmesan, grated

Tomato salad
12 cherry or grape tomatoes,
    halved
1 cup snow pea sprouts, ends
    trimmed
1 large cucumber, cut into small
    chunks
1 ripe avocado, thinly sliced
2 tablespoons fat-free dressing

To serve
4 slices rye bread

1 Whisk together the eggs, milk, dill, salt, and pepper in a bowl.

2 Place 1 teaspoon margarine in each of two small nonstick frying pans. (If you don't have 2 small frying pans, make one large omelet to share.) Heat over medium heat until the margarine starts to bubble. Pour the egg mixture evenly among the two pans and reduce the heat to low. Cook for 2 minutes or until the omelet is almost set.

3 Place half the spinach, salmon, and Parmesan on one side of each omelet. Carefully fold the other side of the omelet over the filling.

4 Meanwhile, to make the salad, place the tomatoes, sprouts, and cucumber in a bowl. Add the dressing and toss gently to combine. Add the avocado.

5 Serve the omelets with the salad and bread.

HAM, CORN, AND ZUCCHINI MUFFINS

*B*est eaten the day they are made, these muffins are an excellent source of fiber.

PREPARATION TIME 20 minutes ■ **COOKING TIME** 20 minutes ■ **MAKES** 6 muffins

PER MUFFIN:

Calories 309

Protein 15 g

Fat 4 g (saturated 1 g)

Carbohydrate 51 g

Fiber 6 g

GI Moderate

GL High

PER SERVING (with salad):

Calories 348

Protein 16 g

Fat 7 g (saturated 2 g)

Carbohydrate 53 g

Fiber 7 g

GI Moderate

GL High

⅔ cup low-fat milk

½ cup low-fat plain yogurt

To serve

4–6 cups mixed salad greens or mesclun

1 red pepper, cut into short, thin strips

1 cup snow peas, cut into long, thin strips

2 tablespoons vinaigrette dressing

1 cup self-rising flour

1 cup whole-wheat self-rising flour

1 teaspoon baking powder

2 tablespoons sugar

1 11-ounce can corn, drained

1 zucchini, coarsely grated

3½ ounces fresh boneless ham, finely chopped

⅓ cup Parmesan, grated

¼ cup fresh chives, chopped

2 eggs

1 Preheat the oven to 400°F and lightly grease a 6-cup muffin pan.

2 Sift the flours and baking powder into a large bowl. Stir in the sugar, corn, zucchini, ham, Parmesan, and chives.

3 Whisk the eggs, milk, and yogurt together. Add to the dry ingredients and use a large metal spoon to mix until just combined. Spoon the mixture evenly into the muffin cups. Bake for 20 minutes or until light golden brown on top and a wooden skewer inserted in the center comes out clean.

4 Meanwhile, combine the salad ingredients. Serve with the warm muffins.

FRIED RICE

The rice for this dish can be cooked and cooled a day ahead. Store in an airtight container in the refrigerator.

PREPARATION TIME 15 minutes (plus cooling time) ■ **COOKING TIME** 25 minutes ■
SERVES 4

PER SERVING:

Calories 460

Protein 32 g

Fat 11.3 g (saturated 3 g)

Carbohydrate 55 g

Fiber 4 g

GI Low

GL High

1¼ cups basmati rice

1 tablespoon olive oil

3 eggs, at room temperature

1 red pepper, finely chopped

½ pound small shrimp, cooked
and peeled

3½ ounces fresh boneless leg
ham, chopped

1 cup peas, frozen

4 shallots, thinly diagonally sliced

1 cup bean sprouts

2 tablespoons low-sodium soy
sauce

1 Cook the rice in a large saucepan of boiling water for 10 to 12 minutes or until tender. Drain well. Spread out in a single layer over two baking trays. Set aside to cool completely.

2 Heat half the oil in a large nonstick wok or frying pan over medium heat. Whisk the eggs until frothy. Pour into the wok or pan and swirl to cover the base. Cook for 2 minutes or until the egg is set. Carefully loosen the edges and turn out onto a cutting board. Set aside to cool. Roll up the omelet and cut into thin strips. Set aside.

3 Heat the remaining oil in the wok over high heat. Add the pepper, shrimp, ham, and peas. Cook, tossing, for 2 minutes. Add the shallots and toss for 1 minute. Add the cooled rice and toss until heated thoroughly. Add the bean sprouts and soy sauce. Toss to combine and serve.

HAM AND VEGETABLE BAKE

*T*his is a terrific recipe for kids—both to make and eat! It is an easy dish that can be eaten hot, warm, or cold, and it is great for picnics, too.

PREPARATION TIME 10 minutes ■ **COOKING TIME** 40 minutes ■ **SERVES** 6

PER SERVING:

Calories 292

Protein 18 g

Fat 10 g (saturated 4 g)

Carbohydrate 30 g

Fiber 6 g

GI Low

GL Low

4 eggs

1 14-ounce can low-sodium
   corn, drained

2 slices fresh boneless ham,
   diced

½ cup cheddar cheese, grated

2 zucchini, grated

2 carrots, grated

1 onion, grated

½ cup whole-wheat self-rising
   flour

1 Preheat the oven to 300°F and grease a 13 x 9-inch pan.

2 Lightly whisk the eggs in a large mixing bowl. Add the corn, ham, cheese, zucchini, carrot, and onion. Gradually, sift in the flour and mix thoroughly to combine.

3 Spoon the mixture into the lasagna dish and press down to flatten the top. Bake for 40 minutes until golden brown and set.

TURKEY AND PEACH SALSA WRAPS

*R*ich in protein and low in fat, these wraps make a delicious and nutritious lunch. Use canned peaches when fresh peaches are not in season—just make sure they are well drained.

PREPARATION TIME 15 minutes ■ **COOKING TIME** none ■ **MAKES** 2 wraps

PER SERVING:

Calories 226

Protein 25 g

Fat 4 g (saturated 1 g)

Carbohydrate 21 g

Fiber 4 g

GI Moderate

GL Moderate

1 peach, peeled and chopped

½ cucumber, chopped

2 teaspoons fresh mint, chopped

1 shallot, sliced

2 whole-wheat tortillas

2 cups iceberg lettuce

5 ounces turkey slices

1 Combine the peach, cucumber, mint, and shallots. Set aside.

2 Lay the tortilla flat and spread the lettuce over two-thirds of the wrap. Arrange the turkey slices over the lettuce.

3 Spoon the peach salsa over the turkey. Roll up to enclose the filling. If not serving immediately, wrap in paper or foil, and store for up to 5 hours. Refrigerate.

TUNA RICE PAPER ROLLS

*I*f you like, use mint instead of coriander in these Vietnamese-style rolls, or leave it out altogether. Plain soy sauce makes a quick dipping sauce if you don't have the other ingredients. A good source of omega-3 fats, these rolls are also high in protein and rich in beta-carotene and vitamin C.

PREPARATION TIME 30 minutes ■ **COOKING TIME** None ■ **MAKES** 12 rolls

PER SERVING:

Calories 160

Protein 24 g

Fat 3 g (saturated 1 g)

Carbohydrate 8 g

Fiber 3 g

GI Moderate

GL Low

12 9-inch round rice paper
   sheets
1 14-ounce can tuna in spring
   water, drained and flaked
1 carrot, grated
2 shallots, finely sliced
2 cups mung bean sprouts
1 red pepper, finely sliced
½ cup coriander leaves

Dipping sauce
1 tablespoon fish sauce
2 tablespoons lime juice
1 tablespoon sweet chili sauce

1 Pour about 2 inches of tepid water into a large shallow dish. Dip one rice paper sheet in the water and soak for about 5 seconds, until just soft and pliable.

2 Drain and pat dry with a paper towel. Place some of the tuna, carrot, shallots, sprouts, pepper, and coriander across one end of the sheet. Fold the end over, then the sides in. Roll up to enclose the filling securely. Repeat with the remaining rice paper sheets and filling ingredients.

3 Combine the fish sauce, lime juice, and chili sauce, and serve with the rolls.

CHICKEN AND RICE SALAD

$\mathcal{T}$his tasty meal is a good source of magnesium, niacin, vitamin C, and vitamin A. Before serving, try scattering some toasted cashew nuts over the top.

PREPARATION TIME 20 minutes ■ **COOKING TIME** 12 minutes ■ **SERVES** 4

PER SERVING:
Calories 312
Protein 21 g
Fat 5 g (saturated 1 g)
Carbohydrate 45 g
Fiber 2 g
GI Moderate
GL Moderate

2 chicken breast fillets, skinless
1 cup basmati rice
1 tablespoon soy sauce
¼ teaspoon sesame oil
1 red pepper, cut into thin strips
1 cup snow peas, sliced
   diagonally
1 carrot, grated
2 shallots, sliced
2 tablespoons lemon juice

1 Gently simmer the chicken in a saucepan of boiling water for 12 minutes, until it is tender and the center of the chicken is no longer pink inside. Remove from pan. When cool enough to handle, cut into thin strips.

2 Meanwhile, cook the rice in a large saucepan of boiling water for about 10 minutes, until tender. Drain, rinse under cold water to stop the cooking, then drain completely.

3 Place the chicken on a plate. Combine the soy sauce and sesame oil and drizzle over the chicken. Toss to coat.

4 Combine the rice and vegetables in a large bowl. Drizzle over the lemon juice and toss to combine. Add the chicken to the rice and mix gently. Serve immediately, or refrigerate until serving time.

LENTIL, BEETS, AND FETA SALAD

PREPARATION TIME 15 minutes ■ **COOKING TIME** none ■ **SERVES** 4

PER SERVING:

Calories 156

Protein 12 g

Fat 5 g (saturated <1 g)

Carbohydrate 12 g

Fiber 5 g

GI Low

GL Low

PER SERVING (with bread):

Calories 264

Protein 16 g

Fat 6 g (saturated 1 g)

Carbohydrate 32 g

Fiber 7 g

GI Low

GL Moderate

1 Combine the lentils, feta, and spinach in a large bowl.

2 Place the lemon juice, oil, and honey in a jar, screw the lid on, and shake until well combined.

3 Drizzle the dressing over the lentil mixture and turn gently to coat.

4 Arrange the lentil mixture on serving plates, and add the beets. Season with salt and pepper, and serve immediately with the bread.

1 14-ounce can lentils, rinsed
   and drained

3½ ounces reduced-fat feta
   cheese, cubed

4 cups baby spinach leaves

1½ tablespoons lemon juice

1 teaspoon extra-virgin olive oil

1 teaspoon honey

1 8-ounce can beets, drained
   and quartered

salt and freshly ground black
   pepper, to taste

4 thick slices sourdough rye
   bread

SWEET POTATO FISH CAKES

PREPARATION TIME 20 minutes (plus chilling time) ■ **COOKING TIME** 15–20 minutes ■ **MAKES** 12 fish cakes

PER SERVING (2 fish cakes with salad):
Calories 214
Protein 21 g
Fat 4 g (saturated <1 g)
Carbohydrate 22 g
Fiber 5 g
GI Low
GL Low

1½ pounds sweet potato, peeled and cut into 1-inch pieces
1¼ pounds boneless whitefish fillets
2 teaspoons olive oil
1 leek, finely chopped
1 red pepper, finely chopped
2 garlic cloves, crushed
2 tablespoons fresh parsley, chopped
salt and freshly ground black pepper, to taste
spray olive oil

To serve
6 cups mixed salad greens or mesclun
1 cucumber, cut into chunks
2 ripe tomatoes, cut into chunks
2 tablespoons fat-free dressing

1 Steam or microwave the sweet potato until tender. Meanwhile, line a steamer basket with non-stick parchment paper. Place the steamer basket over a wok or pan of just-simmering water (make sure the water doesn't touch the basket), cover, and steam the fish for 5 to 10 minutes, until cooked.

2 Heat the oil in a nonstick frying pan over medium heat. Add the leek, pepper, and garlic, and cook, stirring often, for 6 to 7 minutes or until the leek is soft. Set aside.

3 Place the sweet potato in a bowl and mash until smooth. Use a fork to flake the fish into very small pieces. Add the leek mixture, fish, and parsley to the sweet potato and stir well to combine. Season with salt and pepper. Cover and refrigerate until well chilled.

4 Shape the mixture into 12 patties. Place on two baking trays lined with nonstick parchment paper. Refrigerate for 30 minutes. Preheat the oven to 400°F.

5 Spray both sides of the fish cakes lightly with oil. Bake for 15 to 20 minutes or until warmed through and lightly golden. Combine the salad ingredients and serve with the fish cakes.

INDIAN CHICKEN BURGERS

*I*f you like, replace the tikka masala paste with any of your favorite Indian-style pastes. The cooked chicken patties are ideal to take on picnics or to work. Turkish bread can also be used in place of the whole-wheat pita.

PREPARATION TIME 20 minutes ■ **COOKING TIME** 10 minutes ■ **MAKES** 6

PER SERVING (1 patty):
Calories 221
Protein 23 g
Fat 10 g (saturated 2 g)
Carbohydrate 10 g
Fiber 4 g
GI Low
GL Low

PER SERVING (burger):
Calories 460
Protein 32 g
Fat 12 g (saturated 2 g)
Carbohydrate 5 g
Fiber 8 g
GI Moderate
GL High

1¼ pounds chicken breast fillets, skinless, chopped
1 bunch coriander
1 14-ounce can chickpeas, rinsed and drained
1 garlic clove, chopped
2 tablespoons tikka masala paste
2 teaspoons olive oil

To serve
6 whole-wheat pitas, steamed
4–6 cups salad mix
3 small tomatoes, thinly sliced
½ cup low-fat plain yogurt
4½ tablespoons mango chutney

1 Place the chicken, coriander, chickpeas, garlic, and tikka masala paste in a food processor. Process until the mixture is finely chopped and well combined. Shape the mixture into 6 patties. Refrigerate until required.

2 Heat the oil in a large nonstick frying pan over medium heat. Add the chicken patties and cook for 4 to 5 minutes on each side or until cooked through and lightly golden. Meanwhile, split the pita bread open.

3 Top the bases of the bread with the salad mix and tomatoes, then add a chicken patty. Spoon on the yogurt and chutney. Then add the tops of the bread and serve.

Main Dishes

EGGPLANT AND ZUCCHINI PILAF WITH LAMB

PREPARATION TIME 15 minutes ■ **COOKING TIME** 30 minutes ■ **SERVES** 4

PER SERVING:

Calories 496

Protein 30 g

Fat 10 g (saturated 3 g)

Carbohydrate 70 g

Fiber 7 g

GI Moderate

GL High

2 large red peppers, cut into
   1-inch pieces

1 medium eggplant, cut into
   1-inch pieces

2 large zucchini, cut into 1-inch
   pieces

4 teaspoons olive oil

salt and freshly ground black
   pepper, to taste

1 onion, finely chopped

2 garlic cloves, crushed

1½ cups basmati rice, rinsed

2½ cups low-sodium chicken
   broth

4 boneless lamb chops (about 7
   ounces each)

1½ tablespoons fresh parsley,
   finely chopped

1 Preheat the oven to 450°F and line a large roasting pan with nonstick parchment paper.

2 Place the pepper, eggplant, zucchini, and 2 teaspoons of oil in a bowl. Season with salt and pepper and toss well to coat. Spread in a single layer over the lined pan. Bake for 25 to 30 minutes or until very tender and light golden brown.

3 Meanwhile, heat 1 teaspoon of oil in a large, nonstick, heavy-based saucepan over medium heat. Add the onion and garlic and cook, stirring often, for 7 to 8 minutes or until the onion is soft. Increase the heat to high and add the rice. Cook, stirring, for 1 minute. Add the stock, cover, and bring to a boil. Reduce the heat to low and cook, covered, for 10 minutes. Remove from the heat and set aside, covered, for 10 minutes.

4 Brush the lamb with the remaining oil and season with salt and pepper. Preheat a broiler or frying pan over medium-high heat.

Add the lamb and cook for 3 to 4 minutes on each side for medium; or, cook until done to your liking. Set aside for 5 minutes, then slice diagonally.

5 Use a fork to fluff up the rice and separate the grains. Add the roasted vegetables and the parsley to the rice and toss gently to combine.

6 Divide the rice among serving plates and top with the lamb.

MUSHROOM AND VEGETABLE STIR-FRY

PREPARATION TIME 15 minutes ■ **COOKING TIME** 15 minutes ■ **SERVES** 4

PER SERVING:

Calories 335

Protein 9 g

Fat 3 g (saturated <1 g)

Carbohydrate 65 g

Fiber 4 g

GI Moderate

GL High

1½ cups basmati rice

1 bunch baby bok choy

2 teaspoons peanut or vegetable oil

1 small red onion, halved and thinly sliced

1 red pepper, cut into thin strips

½ pound mushrooms, sliced

2 garlic cloves, crushed

2 teaspoons ginger, grated

1 teaspoon red chili, chopped

1 tablespoon low-sodium soy sauce

1 Bring 2¼ cups of water to a boil in a large, tightly covered saucepan. Stir in the rice and quickly replace the lid. Reduce the heat to low and cook for 10 minutes. Remove from heat and let stand, still covered, for 5 minutes.

2 Meanwhile, cut the bok choy in half to separate the leaves from the stems. Cut the leaves into wide shreds and finely slice the stems.

3 Heat the oil in a wok and add the onion. Stir-fry over medium-high heat for 2 minutes, until just tender. Add the pepper and bok choy and stir-fry for 3 minutes.

4 Add the mushrooms, garlic, ginger, and chili, and stir-fry for 3 minutes, until the mushrooms are just soft. Drizzle with soy sauce and toss to combine. Serve immediately with the rice.

SHRIMP AND MANGO SALAD WITH CHILI-LIME DRESSING

This salad is loaded with potassium and is a good source of zinc. The fat it contains is largely monounsaturated. It is best made just before you plan to serve it.

PREPARATION TIME 15 minutes ■ **COOKING TIME** 3 minutes (plus cooling time) ■
SERVES 4

PER SERVING:

Calories 357

Protein 26 g

Fat 13 g (saturated 3 g)

Carbohydrate 31 g

Fiber 7 g

GI Low

GL Moderate

6 small (new) potatoes (about 2½ ounces each), quartered

1½ pounds shrimp, cooked, peeled, and deveined

1 cup snow pea sprouts, ends trimmed

1 cup fresh mint leaves, torn

⅓ cup sweet chili sauce

¼ cup lime juice

1 mango, thinly sliced

1 avocado, thinly sliced

1 Place the potato in a shallow, microwave-safe dish. Pour over about 2 tablespoons of water, cover, and cook on high for 3 minutes or until tender. Set aside to cool.

2 Place the cooled potatoes, shrimp, sprouts, and mint leaves in a bowl and toss to combine.

3 Whisk the chili sauce and lime juice together for the dressing.

4 Divide the salad among serving plates. Top with the mango and avocado slices. Drizzle the dressing on top and serve.

BEEF KEBABS WITH VEGETABLE NOODLE SALAD

*N*ot only is this dish an excellent source of iron and zinc, it also contains vitamin C to enhance absorption of these nutrients. If time permits, you can marinate the meat on skewers overnight.

PREPARATION TIME 20 minutes (plus marinating time) ■
COOKING TIME 10 to 15 minutes ■ **SERVES** 4

PER SERVING:

Calories 408

Protein 36 g

Fat 7 g (saturated 3 g)

Carbohydrate 50 g

Fiber 4 g

GI Low

GL Moderate

1¼ pounds rump steak, lean, cut across the grain into thin strips

16 metal skewers

⅓ cup plum sauce marinade

1 pound Hokkien noodles

1 red pepper, cut into short, thin strips

1 cup snow peas, cut into thin strips

1 cucumber, cut into thin strips

1 bunch coriander

¼ cup low-sodium soy sauce

¼ cup fat-free French dressing

1 Thread the beef strips evenly among the skewers, then place the skewers in a shallow glass or ceramic dish. Pour over the marinade and turn to coat. Set aside for 1 hour to marinate.

2 Preheat a barbecue grill or frying pan over medium heat. Place the noodles in a large heat-proof bowl and cover with boiling water. Set aside for 5 minutes. Drain well, set aside to cool slightly, and then separate the noodles. Add the pepper, snow peas, cucumber, and coriander, and toss to combine.

3 Whisk the soy sauce and dressing together. Add to the salad and toss to combine.

4 Grill the beef skewers for 4 to 6 minutes on each side or until cooked thoroughly. Serve with the noodle salad.

CHICKEN STUFFED WITH SPINACH AND CHEESE

This meal is high in folic acid, niacin, beta-carotene, and fiber.

PREPARATION TIME 15 minute ■ **COOKING TIME** 25–30 minutes ■ **SERVES** 4

PER SERVING:

Calories 498

Protein 55 g

Fat 18 g (saturated 6 g)

Carbohydrate 26 g

Fiber 10 g

GI Low

GL Low

4 chicken breast fillets (about 7 ounces each), skinless

4 slices reduced-fat Swiss cheese (½ ounce each), cut into thin strips

1 cup mushrooms, thinly sliced

2 cups baby spinach leaves

4 wooden toothpicks

2 teaspoons olive oil

salt and freshly ground black pepper, to taste

1⅓ cups Italian tomato sauce

⅓ cup fresh basil leaves, finely shredded

To serve

1 bunch baby carrots, washed

½ pound green beans, trimmed

2 cobs fresh sweet corn, halved

1 Preheat the oven to 350°F. Cut a deep slit (making sure not to cut all the way through) along the length of each chicken breast. Fill each evenly with the cheese, mushrooms, and spinach. Secure the opening with the toothpicks.

2 Heat the oil in a large nonstick frying pan over medium-high heat. Season both sides of the chicken breasts with salt and pepper. Cook for 2 to 3 minutes on each side or until well browned.

3 Transfer the chicken to a shallow ovenproof dish and pour over the tomato sauce. Bake for 15 to 20 minutes, or until the chicken is no longer pink in the center.

4 Meanwhile, steam the carrots, beans, and sweet corn.

5 Remove the toothpicks and place the chicken breasts on serving plates. Pour on the sauce and sprinkle with the basil. Serve with the vegetables.

BARBECUED LAMB WITH LENTIL SALAD AND LEMON-YOGURT DRESSING

PREPARATION TIME 10 minutes (plus marinating time) ■ **COOKING TIME** 15 minutes ■
SERVES 2

PER SERVING:

Calories 447

Protein 49 g

Fat 16 g (saturated 4 g)

Carbohydrate 21 g

Fiber 11 g

GI Low

GL Low

1 tablespoon olive oil

1 clove garlic, crushed

a few sprigs of fresh oregano,
    roughly torn

zest of 1 lemon

2 lamb fillets

Dressing

juice of 1 lemon

½ cup low-fat plain yogurt

salt and freshly ground pepper,
    to taste

Salad

1 tablespoon olive oil

1 14-ounce can lentils, drained

2 medium tomatoes, diced

4 cups baby spinach leaves,
    shredded

1 Combine the olive oil, garlic, oregano, and lemon zest in a bowl. Add the lamb and marinate for at least 30 minutes. Brown the marinated lamb in a frying pan over medium-high heat until just cooked, or longer if you prefer your meat well-done. Remove, cover, and set aside.

2 Meanwhile, combine the lemon juice with the yogurt in a small jar, leaving aside a squeeze of the juice. Season with salt and pepper. Put on the lid and shake to combine.

3 To make the salad, heat the olive oil in a frying pan over medium heat and add the lentils, stirring to warm the lentils thoroughly. Add the tomatoes and spinach and the remaining squeeze of lemon juice, and stir to combine. Remove from heat.

4 Slice the lamb across the grain (about ½ inch thick).

5 Spoon the lentil salad onto serving plates. Top with the sliced meat and pour the dressing over all.

PASTA WITH GRILLED CHICKEN, LEMON, AND BASIL

PREPARATION TIME 15 minutes ■ **COOKING TIME** about 10 minutes ■ **SERVES** 4

PER SERVING:

Calories 494

Protein 30 g

Fat 10 g (saturated 2 g)

Carbohydrate 70 g

Fiber 7 g

GI Low

GL High

2 chicken breast fillets, skinless

spray olive oil

11 ounces pasta, such as penne or spirals

1 cup green peas, fresh or frozen

1 11-ounce can corn, drained

1 tablespoon extra-virgin olive oil

2 tablespoons lemon juice

salt and freshly ground black pepper, to taste

½ cup basil leaves, shredded

1 Spray the chicken lightly with oil and cook on a preheated grill or frying pan for 5 minutes on each side, or until cooked through and the chicken is no longer pink in the center. Cool the chicken slightly, and then tear into bite-sized pieces.

2 Meanwhile, cook the pasta in a large saucepan of boiling salted water according to package directions, or until al dente. Add the peas and corn to the pasta for the last minute of cooking.

3 Drain the pasta, peas, and corn, then return to the pan. Drizzle with the extra-virgin olive oil and lemon juice, and add the torn chicken pieces. Season well with salt and pepper, then toss to combine.

4 Spoon onto serving plates and top with the basil leaves. Serve immediately.

THAI–STYLE TOFU AND NOODLE SOUP

*A*n excellent source of folic acid and vitamin C and a good source of calcium, magnesium, and potassium, this soup is a meal in itself. The tofu doesn't need cooking, but adding it in at the beginning helps it absorb the flavors. Lemongrass is available either fresh or in jars from large supermarkets. Choose fresh if you can, for the best flavor. Mung bean vermicelli, sometimes called cellophane noodles or bean thread vermicelli, is available in the Asian food section of supermarkets.

PREPARATION TIME 20 minutes ■ **COOKING TIME** about 5 minutes ■ **SERVES** 4

PER SERVING:
Calories 220
Protein 16 g
Fat 7 g (saturated 1 g)
Carbohydrate 21 g
Fiber 7 g
GI Low
GL Low

3½ ounces mung bean vermicelli

4 cups vegetable stock

1 tablespoon lemongrass, finely chopped

1½ teaspoons grated ginger

1½ teaspoons red chili pepper, finely chopped

1 pound firm tofu, cut into ½-inch cubes

1 bunch asparagus, cut into 2-inch lengths

1 small head broccoli, cut into small florets

12 baby ears of corn, cut in half lengthways and crossways

2 shallots, finely sliced

fresh coriander leaves, to serve

1 Place the vermicelli in a large heat-proof bowl and cover with boiling water. Let stand for 10 minutes.

2 Meanwhile, pour the vegetable stock into a large saucepan. Add the lemongrass, ginger, chili, and tofu. Bring to a boil.

3 Add the asparagus, broccoli, and corn. Return to a boil, then cook for 2 minutes.

4 Drain the noodles, then divide between four serving bowls and top with the vegetables, tofu, and stock. Sprinkle each bowl with shallots and coriander leaves and serve immediately.

HERBED FISH PARCELS WITH SWEET POTATO WEDGES AND COLESLAW

*H*igh in protein and low in fat, this meal is a far cry from fish and chips. It's also loaded with beta-carotene, potassium, and magnesium.

PREPARATION TIME 30 minutes ■ **COOKING TIME** 40 minutes ■ **SERVES** 4

PER SERVING:

Calories 279

Protein 34 g

Fat 8 g (saturated 1 g)

Carbohydrate 22 g

Fiber 5 g

GI Low

GL Low

1¼ pounds sweet potato, peeled
and cut into wedges

spray olive oil

1 teaspoon Cajun spice mix

4 whitefish fillets (about 5 ounces
each)

2 teaspoons dill, chopped

2 teaspoons lemon rind, finely
grated

freshly ground black pepper, to
taste

Coleslaw

3 cups cabbage, finely shredded

1 carrot, grated

½ red onion, finely chopped

¼ cup Italian parsley, chopped

1 tablespoon canola mayonnaise

2 tablespoons lemon juice

1 Preheat the oven to 400°F and line a large baking tray with non-stick parchment paper.

2 Spray the sweet potato wedges lightly with oil, and sprinkle with the Cajun spice mix. Toss to coat. Arrange in a single layer on the lined tray, and bake for 25 minutes.

3 Meanwhile, tear 4 squares of nonstick parchment paper. Place a fish fillet on each sheet and sprinkle with the dill and lemon rind. Season with pepper. Fold and wrap the parchment paper securely to enclose the fish, and then place on a baking tray. Transfer to the oven and bake for 15 minutes (so the sweet potatoes cook for 40 minutes total).

4 For the coleslaw, combine the cabbage, carrot, onion, and parsley in a large bowl. Add the mayonnaise and lemon juice; toss to combine. Serve the coleslaw with the fish and wedges.

MOROCCAN-STYLE LENTIL AND VEGETABLE STEW WITH COUSCOUS

*T*his meal is a great source of fiber and is rich in vitamin C and folic acid.

PREPARATION TIME 25 minutes ■ **COOKING TIME** 50 minutes ■ **SERVES** 4

PER SERVING:

Calories 276

Protein 14 g

Fat 3 g (saturated <1 g)

Carbohydrate 44 g

Fiber 8 g

GI Moderate

GL High

2 teaspoons olive oil

1 onion, chopped

2 cloves garlic, crushed

2 teaspoons grated ginger

2 teaspoons ground cumin

2 teaspoons ground coriander

1 cup vegetable stock

1 14-ounce can chopped tomatoes

1 small head cauliflower, cut into small florets

1 small eggplant, cut into 1-inch cubes

1½ cups green beans, cut into 2-inch lengths

1 14-ounce can lentils, rinsed and drained

1 cup couscous

1 Heat the oil in a large saucepan over medium heat. Add the onion and cook for 5 minutes until soft and lightly golden. Add the garlic, ginger, and spices and cook for 30 seconds, stirring.

2 Add the stock and tomatoes. Stir to combine, scraping the bottom of the pan. Add the cauliflower, eggplant, and beans, stir to combine, and bring to a boil. Reduce the heat to medium-low and simmer, covered, for 30 minutes, until the vegetables are tender. Uncover and cook for 10 minutes longer.

3 Stir in the lentils and cook for 5 minutes to heat thoroughly.

4 Meanwhile, bring 1¼ cups of water to the boil in a medium-size saucepan. Add the couscous, cover tightly, and turn off the heat. Let stand for 5 minutes, then uncover and fluff up the grains with a fork.

5 Serve the spicy vegetable stew over the couscous.

Snacks and
Sweet Treats

HERBED SALMON SPREAD

This spread is rich in omega-3 fats and delicious with whole-grain crackers or low-GI bread. If you prefer, you could replace the salmon with tuna. It will keep in the refrigerator for up to three days.

PREPARATION TIME 10 minutes ■ **COOKING TIME** none ■ **SERVES** 4

PER SERVING:

Calories 150

Protein 15 g

Fat 10 g (saturated 4 g)

Carbohydrate 1 g

Fiber <1 g

GI Low

GL Low

1 Place the salmon in a bowl and flake with a fork. Add the ricotta, lemon rind and juice, and herbs. Mash with a fork until well combined.

2 Season to taste.

1 7-ounce can salmon (red or
    pink) in spring water, drained

7 ounces reduced-fat ricotta

½ teaspoon lemon rind, finely
    grated

2 teaspoons lemon juice

1 tablespoon chives, chopped

1 tablespoon Italian parsley,
    chopped

salt and freshly ground black
    pepper, to taste

BRUSCHETTA WITH BASIL AND TOMATOES

PREPARATION TIME 10 minutes ■ **COOKING TIME** about 5 minutes ■ **MAKES** 4

PER SERVING:

Calories 101

Protein 4 g

Fat 1 g (saturated <1 g)

Carbohydrate 18 g

Fiber 3 g

GI Low

GL Low

4 slices sourdough bread (preferably day-old)

1 garlic clove, peeled and halved

2 medium tomatoes, diced

½ small red onion, finely chopped

¼ cup basil leaves, shredded

1 teaspoon balsamic vinegar (optional)

salt and freshly ground pepper, to taste

1 Toast the bread on both sides until golden brown. Rub with the cut garlic clove and set aside to cool.

2 Combine the tomatoes with the onion and basil. Drizzle with the balsamic vinegar (optional) and season with salt and pepper.

3 Spoon the tomato mixture onto the sourdough toast slices and serve immediately.

EGGPLANT AND BEAN PURÉE

𝒯his eggplant purée is a nutritious and tasty addition to sandwiches, or can be enjoyed spread on whole-grain crackers or whole-grain pita bread.

PREPARATION TIME 20 minutes ■ **COOKING TIME** 40 minutes (plus cooling time) ■
SERVES 6

PER SERVING:
Calories 61
Protein 5 g
Fat 3 g (saturated <1 g)
Carbohydrate 3 g
Fiber 4 g
GI Low
GL Low

PER SERVING
(with vegetables):
Calories 75
Protein 5 g
Fat 3 g (saturated <1 g)
Carbohydrate 6 g
Fiber <1 g
GI Low
GL Low

1 Preheat the oven to 375°F and line a baking tray with lightly oiled foil.

2 Place the eggplant cut side down on the foil. Bake for 35 minutes, until the eggplant is soft.

3 Cool the eggplant until just warm, then scoop the flesh out of the skin and place in a food processor. Add the soybeans, cumin, garlic, and lemon juice, and process until smooth.

4 Serve with the vegetables for dipping.

1 large eggplant, cut in half
   lengthwise
1 14-ounce can soybeans, rinsed
   and drained
1 teaspoon ground cumin
1 clove garlic, crushed
2 tablespoons lemon juice
1 red pepper, cut into sticks
1 cucumber, cut into rounds
1 carrot, cut into sticks

APRICOT AND ALMOND COOKIES

*T*hese cookies will keep in an airtight container for three to four days.

PREPARATION TIME 15 minutes ■ **COOKING TIME** 15 minutes ■
MAKES about 16 cookies

PER COOKIE:

Calories 90

Protein 2 g

Fat 4 g (saturated <1 g)

Carbohydrate 13 g

Fiber 1 g

GI Low

GL Low

3½ ounces dried apricots, diced
3½ ounces ground almonds
½ cup sugar
⅓ cup plain, all-purpose flour
2 egg whites, at room temperature

1 Preheat the oven to 325°F and line two baking trays with non-stick parchment paper.

2 Place the apricots, almonds, sugar, and flour in a bowl and mix well to combine.

3 Whisk the egg whites until frothy. Add to the apricot mixture and mix until well combined.

4 Use slightly wet hands to shape tablespoonfuls of the mixture into balls. Place on the lined trays and use a spoon to press out slightly.

5 Bake for 12 to 15 minutes until the cookies are set and lightly golden on the bottom. Let cool on the trays for 5 minutes before transferring to a wire rack to cool completely.

MUESLI AND HONEY SLICE

This slice will keep in an airtight container for three to four days.

PREPARATION TIME 10 minutes ■ **COOKING TIME** 20 to 25 minutes ■
MAKES 16 pieces

PER SERVING:

Calories 153

Protein 3 g

Fat 7 g (saturated 1 g)

Carbohydrate 21 g

Fiber 2 g

GI Low

GL Low

½ cup pure honey

7 tablespoons canola margarine

2 eggs

2 cups natural muesli

½ cup self-rising flour

1 Preheat the oven to 325°F and line a 6-inch x 6-inch baking pan with nonstick parchment paper.

2 Place the honey and margarine in a small saucepan. Stir over low heat until the margarine melts and the mixture is well combined. Set aside to cool. Pour into a bowl and whisk in the eggs.

3 Combine the muesli and flour in a bowl. Add the cooled honey mixture and stir well to combine. Pour into the lined pan and smooth the surface. Bake for 20 to 25 minutes or until set and golden. Set aside in the pan to cool.

4 Cut the slice into 16 pieces. Store in an airtight container.

BANANA AND RICOTTA TOAST

PREPARATION TIME 5 minutes ■ **COOKING TIME** 5 minutes ■ **MAKES** 4 toasts

PER SERVING:

Calories 171

Protein 6 g

Fat 3 g (saturated 2 g)

Carbohydrate 29 g

Fiber 3 g

GI Low

GL Moderate

1 Use electric beaters to beat the ricotta, honey, and cinnamon until almost smooth.

2 Toast the bread until golden.

3 Spread the ricotta mixture evenly on the bread. Top with the bananas. Drizzle over a little honey and an extra sprinkle of cinnamon and serve immediately.

3½ ounces low-fat fresh ricotta

1 tablespoon pure honey

pinch of ground cinnamon

4 slices whole-grain bread

2 small bananas, diagonally sliced

extra honey, to serve

extra cinnamon, to serve

FRUIT PARFAITS

*T*he almond bread referred to is a very thin, sweet cookie, similar to Italian biscotti, but wafer-thin. It's available from the cookie or gourmet section of your supermarket.

PREPARATION TIME 20 minutes ■ **REFRIGERATION TIME** 30 minutes ■ **MAKES** 4 parfaits

PER SERVING:

Calories 256

Protein 12 g

Fat 4 g (saturated <1 g)

Carbohydrate 38 g

Fiber 4 g

GI Low

GL Moderate

1 cup fresh raspberries
1 tablespoon orange juice
3 ounces almond bread or
   biscotti
4 nectarines or peaches, sliced
2 cups low-fat vanilla yogurt

1 Place the raspberries in a bowl, then add the orange juice. Mash with a fork, and stir to make a chunky sauce.

2 Break the almond bread into bite-sized pieces. Layer the nectarines (or peaches), raspberry sauce, almond bread, and yogurt in parfait glasses.

3 To let the flavors blend, refrigerate the parfaits for 30 minutes before serving.

BLUEBERRY CHEESECAKES

PREPARATION TIME 20 minutes ▪ **REFRIGERATION TIME** 1 hour ▪ **MAKES** 4 cheesecakes

PER SERVING:

Calories 206

Protein 10 g

Fat 13 g (saturated 5 g)

Carbohydrate 12 g

Fiber 2 g

GI Low

GL Low

10 ounces low-fat ricotta

1 tablespoon pure honey

1 teaspoon finely grated orange rind

1 cup fresh blueberries

⅓ cup walnuts, finely chopped

4 strawberries, sliced

1 Line four ½-cup-capacity ramekins with plastic wrap.

2 Place the ricotta, honey, and orange rind in a bowl and mash with a fork.

3 Combine two-thirds of the blueberries with the ricotta mixture and divide between the ramekins. Press in firmly and smooth the surface.

4 Sprinkle the walnuts on top. Smooth out with the back of a spoon and press the nuts into the mixture. Refrigerate for 1 hour to form and chill.

5 To serve, invert onto a plate and peel away the plastic wrap. Top each cake with a sliced strawberry and serve with the remaining blueberries.

CREAMED RICE WITH RHUBARB AND STRAWBERRIES

𝒯here is almost no fat in this dessert. The rhubarb mixture will keep in an airtight container in the refrigerator for three to four days.

PREPARATION TIME 10 minutes (plus cooling time) ■ **COOKING TIME** 25 minutes ■ **SERVES** 4

PER SERVING:

Calories 242

Protein 8 g

Fat 0 g

Carbohydrate 50 g

Fiber 4 g

GI Low

GL High

1 bunch rhubarb, ends trimmed and cut into 1¼-inch pieces
¼ cup sugar
2 cups strawberries, hulled and halved
½ cup cooked basmati rice
2 tablespoons sugar, plus a little extra
2 cups skim milk
pinch of ground cinnamon

1 Place the rhubarb and sugar in a medium-size, heavy-based saucepan. Stir constantly over medium heat for 5 minutes until the rhubarb starts to soften. Add the strawberries and cook for 5 minutes longer or until the rhubarb and strawberries are tender. Remove from the heat and set aside to cool.

2 Meanwhile, place the rice, extra sugar, and 1¼ cups of the skim milk in another medium-size, heavy-based saucepan. Stir over low heat until the sugar dissolves, then increase the heat and bring to a simmer. Reduce the heat to low, cover, and cook for 12 minutes.

3 Remove from the heat and stir in the remaining milk, then cover and set aside for 10 minutes. Stir in a pinch of cinnamon and serve with the rhubarb mixture.

ORANGE AND PASSION FRUIT MOUSSE

This dessert is a good source of calcium and phosphorus and contains less than 1 gram of fat per serving. It will keep in the refrigerator for up to two days.

PREPARATION TIME 15 minutes ■ **COOKING TIME** 2 minutes
(plus chilling and setting time) ■ **SERVES** 6

PER SERVING:

Calories 119

Protein 7 g

Fat <1 g (saturated <1 g)

Carbohydrate 23 g

Fiber 1 g

GI Low

GL Low

⅔ cup freshly squeezed orange juice

⅓ cup sugar

2 teaspoons powdered gelatin

⅓ cup fresh passion fruit pulp

1½ cups light evaporated milk, chilled

extra passion fruit, to serve (optional)

1 Place the orange juice and sugar in a small saucepan. Heat until hot, not boiling. Remove from heat and stir in the gelatin until it dissolves. Pour the mixture into a small heat-proof bowl and set aside to cool slightly. Stir in the passion fruit pulp.

2 In a large bowl, use electric beaters to whisk the evaporated milk until light and fluffy. Add the orange mixture and stir to combine. Cover the bowl and chill for 1 to 1½ hours, stirring often, or until the mousse starts to thicken and set slightly. (Stirring will help the passion fruit to suspend in the mousse rather than sinking to the bottom.)

3 Spoon the mousse mixture into individual serving dishes. Refrigerate for 3 to 4 hours longer, or until set.

4 Serve the mousse topped with extra passion fruit, if desired.

PART FIVE

The GI Table

A NOTE ABOUT THE TABLE

The following table gives a comprehensive, up-to-date listing of the GI values of hundreds of popular foods in alphabetical order along with our suggestions for how freely you should eat each food.

The table will help you to select lower-GI varieties in each food category and therefore enable you to lower the GI of your overall diet.

Some foods contain very little or no carbohydrate and, as a result, do not give a glycemic response when eaten. These foods are marked with this symbol ★ and do not have a GI value. We have nevertheless given these foods a recommendation (or otherwise) for their role in the Low GI Diet Revolution.

Foods marked with the ▼ symbol may be high in saturated fat. We recommend that you check the food label for saturated fat content and limit your intake of foods for which saturated fat accounts for more than 20 percent of the total fat content. With fresh foods, such as meat and seafood, remove visible fat and prepare using small amounts of polyunsaturated or monounsaturated fats if desired.

If you see the symbol ✣ next to a GI value, this means that the value is an average result for that particular food. The average may be of ten studies or of only two to four studies.

Not all foods have had their GI values measured. This list, therefore, although extensive, is not complete. If you don't see a GI value for a food or drink you're looking up, then contact the manufacturer to ask them if they have had this product's GI value tested. Not all food manufacturers are aware of GI testing yet, and some might have GI values for their products, but do not allow them to be published.

The GI values in the table are correct at the time of publication. However, the formulation of commercial foods can change, and the GI might be altered. You can rely on those foods showing the GI symbol (see page 98). You will find revised and new data on our Web site, www.glycemicindex.com.

FOOD	GI VALUE	
Alfalfa sprouts	★	An everyday food
All-Bran, breakfast cereal, Kellogg's	34⠇	An excellent choice
All-Bran Fruit 'n' Oats, breakfast cereal, Kellogg's	39	An excellent choice
Angel food cake, plain	67▼	Okay now and again
Apple, fresh	38⠇	Great anytime
Apple, dried	29	Great for snacks—in moderate amounts

APPLE JUICE

Apple juice, no added sugar	40⠇	
Apple juice, clear, no added sugar	44	
Apple juice, cloudy, no added sugar	37	Enjoy in moderation—
Apple and blackcurrant juice, pure	45	about one glass a day
Apple and cherry juice, pure	43	
Apple and mandarin juice, pure	53	
Apple and mango juice, pure	47	
Apple muffin, home-made	46▼	Now and then—GI varies with each recipe
Apricot-filled fruit bar, whole-wheat pastry	50▼	Okay for an occasional snack
Apricot fruit spread, reduced sugar	55	Enjoy in moderation
Apricots, canned in light syrup	64	Go easy—fresh is best
Apricots, dried	30	A nutritious snack or addition to meals
Apricots, fresh	57	Great anytime
Arborio, risotto rice, white, boiled	69	A fair choice
Artichokes, globe, fresh or canned in brine	★	An everyday food
Asparagus	★	An everyday food
Avocado	★	Good fat, eat in moderation
Bagel, white	72	Take it easy
Baked beans, canned in tomato sauce	49⠇	A healthy convenience food
Banana, raw	52⠇	Everyday food—the less ripe, the lower the GI
Banana cake, home-made	51⠇▼	Go easy—GI varies with recipe; energy dense
Banana smoothie drink, low-fat	30	A low-fat snack or light meal
Barley, pearled, boiled	25⠇	A star performer—very low GI
Barley, rolled, raw	66	Fiber rich, has a lower GI when served as porridge
Basmati rice, white, boiled	58	A good choice
Bean curd, tofu, plain, unsweetened	★	An excellent source of lean protein
Bean sprouts, raw	★	An everyday food

BEANS Natural super foods—low GI and nutritious

Black, boiled	30	
Black-eyed peas, soaked, boiled	42	Natural super foods—
Butter, canned, drained	36	low GI and nutritious
Butter, dried, boiled	31⠇	
Cannellini	31	

⠇ average   ★ little or no carbs   ▼ high in saturated fat

FOOD	GI VALUE	
Dark red kidney, canned, drained	43	
Four bean mix, canned, drained	37	
Green	★	
Lima, baby, frozen, reheated	32	
Mung	39	Natural super foods—
Navy, cooked, canned	38÷	low GI and nutritious
Navy, dried, boiled	33÷	
Pinto, canned, drained	45	
Pinto, dried, boiled	39	
Red kidney, canned, drained	36	
Soy, canned, drained	14÷	
Soy, dried, boiled	18	
Beef	▼★	Eat it lean
Beer, (4.6% alcohol)	66	Go slow—drink in moderation, if at all
Beets, canned	64	A good source of antioxidants
Berry Bliss Nutrition Bar	22	Snack bar
Blueberry muffin, commercially made	59▼	Occasional treat
Bok choy	★	An everyday food
Bran Flakes, breakfast cereal, Kellogg's	74	Go slow
Bran muffin, commercially made	60▼	Now and then
BREAD		
Bagel, white	72	
Black rye bread	76	
Dark rye bread	86	
Gluten-free multigrain bread	79	
Hamburger bun, white	61	
Kaiser rolls, white	73	
Lebanese bread, white	75	
Multigrain 9 grain bread	43	
Multigrain sandwich bread	65	
Oat bran and honey bread	49	Choose lower GI varieties for
Pita bread, white	57	everyday eating
Pumpernickel bread	50÷	
Raisin bread, whole grain	44	
Regular, sliced white bread, enriched	71	
Seeded rye bread	51	
Sourdough rye bread	48	
Sourdough wheat bread	54	
Soy and linseed bread	36	
Spelt multigrain bread	54	
Stone-ground whole-wheat bread	59	
White sandwich bread	70	
Whole-wheat, enriched wheat flour	70	
Wonder White, white bread	80	

÷ average   ★ little or no carbs   ▼ high in saturated fat

FOOD	GI VALUE	
BREAKFAST CEREALS		
—All-Bran, Kellogg's	34⊹	
—All-Bran Fruit 'n' Oats, Kellogg's	39	
Bran Flakes, Kellogg's	74	
Coco Pops, Kellogg's	77⊹	
Corn Flakes, Kellogg's	77	
Corn Pops, Kellogg's	80	
Crunchy Nut Corn Flakes, Kellogg's	72	
Fruit Loops, Kellogg's	69	
Frosted Flakes, Kellogg's	55	
Golden Grahams, General Mills	71	
Hi-Bran Weet-Bix, regular	61	
Honey Smacks, Kellogg's	71	
Mini Wheats, Kellogg's	72	
Mini Wheats, Wholewheat, Kellogg's	58	
Muesli, gluten-free, with 1.5% fat milk	39	
Muesli, low-fat	54	Choose lower GI varieties
Muesli, natural	49⊹	for everyday eating
Muesli, Swiss, Alpen	55	
Nutri-Grain, Kellogg's	66	
Oat bran, raw, unprocessed	55⊹	
Oat Bran Weet-Bix	57	
Oats, rolled, raw	59	
Oatmeal, instant, made with water	82	
Oatmeal, made from steel-cut oats with water	52	
Oatmeal, regular, made from old-fashioned rolled oats with water	51	
Porridge, Multi-grain, made with water	55	
Puffed buckwheat	65	
Puffed Wheat	80	
Rice Bran, Extruded	19	
Rice Krispies, breakfast cereal, Kellogg's	82	
Semolina, cooked	55⊹	
Shredded Wheat	75⊹	
Special K, regular, Kellogg's	56	
Raisin Bran Flakes, Kellogg's	73	
BREAKFAST CEREAL BARS		
Crunchy Nut Corn Flakes Bar, Kellogg's	72	Now and then; choose lower GI,
Kudos Whole Grain Bar, chocolate chip	62	lower saturated fat varieties
Nutrigrain Fruit Bar	57	
Breton wheat crackers	67▼	Go slow
Broad beans	79	No problem in moderation
Broccoli	★	An everyday food

⊹ average   ★ little or no carbs   ▼ high in saturated fat

FOOD	GI VALUE	
Broken rice, white, cooked in rice cooker	86	Take it easy
Brussels sprouts	★	An everyday food
Buckwheat, boiled	54÷	A nutritious alternative to rice
Buckwheat, pancakes, gluten-free, packet mix	102	Go slow
Bulgur, cracked wheat, ready to eat	48÷	Delicious in salads such as tabbouli
Bun, hamburger, white	61	Eat in moderation—use grainy rolls instead
Butter beans, canned, drained	36	A great choice
Butter beans, dried, boiled	31÷	super food
Cabbage	★	An everyday food
CAKES		
Angel food cake, plain	67▼	
Banana cake, home-made	51÷▼	
Chocolate cake, made from packet mix with frosting, Betty Crocker	38▼	
Cupcake with strawberry icing, commercial	73▼	Take it easy—indulgence foods
Pound cake, plain	54▼	
Sponge cake, plain, unfilled	46▼	
Vanilla cake, made from packet mix with vanilla frosting, Betty Crocker	42▼	
Calamari rings, squid, not battered or crumbed	★	Try prepared with unsaturated fats
Cannellini beans	31	A five-star food
Cantaloupe, fresh	67÷	Eat in moderation
Capellini pasta, white, boiled	45	Good choice; watch portion size
Carrot juice, freshly made	43	Go for it
Carrots, peeled, boiled	41÷	An everyday food
Cashew nuts, salted	22	A great snack, in moderation—best unsalted
Cauliflower	★	An everyday food
Celery	★	Whenever you like
Cheese	▼★	Energy dense; best in small amounts
Cheese-flavored snack	74▼	Indulgence food
Cheese tortellini, cooked	50▼	In moderation
Cherries, dark, raw	63	Enjoy in moderation
Chicken	▼★	Eat it lean without skin
Chicken nuggets, frozen, reheated in microwave 5 min	46▼	Go slow
Chickpeas, canned in brine	40	A convenient and nutritious food
Chickpeas, dried, boiled	28÷	One of nature's super foods
Chilies, fresh or dried	★	An everyday food
Chives, fresh	★	An everyday food
CHOCOLATE		
Cadbury's Milk Chocolate, plain	49▼	
Dark chocolate, plain, regular	41÷▼	Indulgence food—energy dense
Dove, milk chocolate	45▼	

÷ average　　★ little or no carbs　　▼ high in saturated fat

FOOD	GI VALUE	
Mars Bar, regular	62▼	
Milk, plain, Nestlé	42▼	
Milk, plain, reduced sugar	35▼	
Milk, plain, regular	41❖▼	Indulgence food—energy dense
Milk, plain, with fructose instead of regular sugar	20▼	
Milky Bar, white, Nestlé	44▼	
Snickers Bar, regular	41▼	
Chocolate cake, made from packet mix with frosting, Betty Crocker	38▼	Special occasion food
Chocolate Charger Nutrition Bar	28	snack bar
Chocolate hazelnut smoothie drink, low-fat	34	Enjoy in moderation
Chocolate hazelnut spread, Nutella	30	Enjoy in moderation
Chocolate mousse, diet, Nestlé	37	A good choice for a snack or dessert
Chocolate mousse, Nestlé	37	Enjoy in moderation
Chocolate pudding, instant, made from packet with whole milk	47❖▼	Go slow—use low-fat milk
Coca-Cola, soft drink	63	An occasional treat
Coco Pops, breakfast cereal, Kellogg's	77	An occasional treat
Coffee, black, no milk or sugar	★	Drink in moderation
Condensed milk, sweetened, full fat	61▼	Go slow
Consommé, clear, chicken or vegetable	★	A nice light entrée
COOKIES		
Arrowroot	63▼	
Digestives, gluten-free	58▼	
Digestives, regular	59❖▼	
Graham wafers, plain	74▼	Indulgence foods—limit your intake
Oatmeal	54▼	
Rich Tea	55▼	
Shortbread, plain	64▼	
Vanilla wafer, plain	77▼	
Cordial, orange, reconstituted	66	Okay in moderation
Corn, sweet, on the cob, boiled 20 min	48	A good choice—take it easy with the butter
Corn chips, plain, salted	42▼	Take care—low GI due to high fat content
Corn Flakes, breakfast cereal, Kellogg's	77	Now and then
Corn Flakes, Crunchy Nut, breakfast cereal, Kellogg's	72	Use as a special treat
Cornmeal (polenta), boiled	68	Enjoy in moderation
Corn pasta, gluten-free, boiled	78	Serve al dente for a lower GI
Corn Pops, breakfast cereal, Kellogg's	80	Go slow
Couscous, boiled 5 min	65❖	Eat in moderation
CRACKERS AND CRISPBREADS		
Breton wheat crackers	67▼	Now and then—choose lower GI, lower saturated fat types
Corn Thins, gluten-free, puffed corn cakes	87	
Kavli Norwegian Crispbread	71	

❖ average   ★ little or no carbs   ▼ high in saturated fat

FOOD	GI VALUE	
Plain salted crackers	55▼	Now and then—choose lower GI, lower saturated fat types
Puffed rice cakes, white	82	
Ryvita crispbread	69	
Water cracker, plain	71÷	
Cranberries, dried, sweetened snacks	64	Good for cooking and occasional
Cranberry Juice Cocktail, Ocean Spray	52	Enjoy in moderation
Crème Caramel, Diet, Nestlé	33	A good choice for desert
Crispix, breakfast cereal	87	Go slow
Croissant, plain	67▼	Indulgence food
Crumpet, white	69	Enjoy in moderation
Crunchy Nut Corn Flakes Bar, Kellogg's	72	Indulgence food
Crunchy Nut Corn Flakes, breakfast cereal, Kellogg's	72	An occasional treat
Cucumber	★	An everyday food
Cupcake, strawberry-iced, commercial	73▼	Go slow
Custard, home-made from milk	43▼	Okay occasionally—use low-fat milk wheat starch and sugar
Custard, vanilla, reduced-fat	37	Good with fruit as a dessert
Custard apple, fresh, flesh only	54	Great anytime
Dark rye bread	86	Take it easy
Dates, dried	39	Great anytime
Diet jelly	★	A low calorie alternative to regular jelly
Diet soft drinks	★	Low in calories and nutrients—enjoy in moderation
Dried apple	29	Great for snacks—in moderate amounts
Duck	▼★	Serve the meat lean without skin
Eggplant	★	An everyday food
Eggs	▼★	Nutritious; use unsaturated fat in cooking
Endive	★	An everyday food
Ensure, vanilla drink	48	A nutrition supplement
Fanta, orange soft drink	68	An occasional treat
Fat-free yogurts, with sugar	40÷	A good choice
Fennel	★	An everyday food
Fermented probiotic milk drink	46	A nutrition supplement
Fettuccine, egg, cooked	32	The GI will increase if overcooked
Figs, dried	61	A nutritious snack now and then
Fish	★	A fantastic food—prepare with minimal fat
Fish fingers	38▼	Go slow—low GI due to fat content
Four bean mix, canned, drained	37	An everyday food
French fries, frozen, reheated in microwave	75▼	Take it easy
French vanilla ice-cream, premium	38▼	Indulgence food
Fruit Loops, breakfast cereal	69	Take it easy

÷ average   ★ little or no carbs   ▼ high in saturated fat

FOOD	GI VALUE	
Frosted Flakes, Kellogg's	55	An occasional treat
Fructose, pure	19⋅❖	Powdered sugar that naturally occurs in fruit
FRUIT, CANNED		
Apricots, in light syrup	64	
Fruit cocktail	55	
Peach, in heavy syrup	58	Enjoy the fruit, avoid the syrup (it's energy dense)
Peach, in light syrup	57⋅❖	
Peach, in natural juice	45	
Pear, in natural juice	44⋅❖	
FRUIT, DRIED		
Apple	29	
Apricots	31⋅❖	
Cranberries, sweetened	64	Nutritious, but concentrated— enjoy in moderation
Dates, pitted	103	
Figs, dried	61	
Prunes, pitted	29	
Raisins	64	
FRUIT, FRESH		
Apple	38⋅❖	
Apricots	57	
Banana	52⋅❖	
Cantaloupe	67⋅❖	
Cherries, dark	63	All fruit is rich in antioxidants and nutrients—a high GI should not deter you
Grapefruit	25	
Grapes	53⋅❖	
Kiwi fruit	53	
Mango	51⋅❖	
Montmorency Frozen Tart Cherries	54	
Orange	42⋅❖	
Papaya	56	
Fruit cocktail, canned fruit	55	Fresh fruit salad is a better choice
Fruit Fingers, Heinz Kidz, banana	61	Okay occasionally
FRUIT JUICE		
Apple, clear, no added sugar	44	
Apple, cloudy, no added sugar	37	
Apple, no added sugar	40⋅❖	
Apple and blackcurrant, pure	45	
Apple and cherry, pure	43	Enjoy in small amounts— eating fresh fruit is much more satiating
Apple and mandarin, pure	53	
Apple and mango, pure	47	
Carrot, freshly made	43	
Cranberry Juice Cocktail, Ocean Spray	52	
Grapefruit, unsweetened	48	

❖ average ★ little or no carbs ▼ high in saturated fat

FOOD	GI VALUE	
Orange, unsweetened, fresh	50÷	Enjoy in small amounts—eating fresh fruit is much more satiating
Orange, unsweetened, from concentrate	53	
Pineapple, unsweetened	46	
Tomato, no added sugar	38	
Fruit and Nut Bar	56	A reasonable snack
Garlic	★	An everyday food
Gatorade sports drink	78	Beverage for serious sports people
Gelati, sucrose-free, chocolate	37	Low GI, low-fat dessert
Gelati, sucrose-free, vanilla	39	Low GI, low-fat dessert
Ginger	★	An everyday food
Glucose tablets	100	A dietary supplement—use with care
GLUTEN-FREE PRODUCTS ⅂ Gluten-free alternatives for common carb-rich foods		
Buckwheat pancake mix, ready to eat	102	
Corn pasta, boiled	78	Avoid overcooking, so GI doesn't rise further
Muesli with 1.5% fat milk	39	A great gluten-free breakfast choice
Multigrain bread	79	Has more fiber than white gluten-free bread
Rice and corn pasta	76	Look for protein-enriched varieties
Spaghetti, in tomato sauce	68	A fair choice
Split pea and soy pasta shells, boiled	29	
Glutinous rice, white, cooked in rice cooker	98	Go slow
Gnocchi, cooked	68	A fair choice
Golden syrup	63	An occasional treat
Golden Grahams, General Mills	71	Now and then
Grape nectar	52	A substitute for honey—use in moderation
Grapefruit, fresh	25	An everyday food
Grapefruit juice, unsweetened	48	Drink in moderation
Grapes, fresh	53÷	An everyday food
Green beans	★	Any time you like
Green pea soup, canned	66	A fair choice
Gummi confectionery, based on glucose syrup	94÷	Go slow—an occasional treat
Ham, leg or shoulder	▼★	Use lean cuts and eat in moderation
Hamburger bun, white	61	Take it easy
Heinz Baked Beans in tomato sauce, canned	51	A good choice
Herbs, fresh or dried	★	An everyday food
Hi-Bran Weet-Bix, regular	61	A lower GI version of Weet-Bix
HONEY Pure, 100%	55÷	Best used in moderation—the lower GI types are pure floral honeys, look for them at health food shops, markets, and orchards
Honey Smacks, breakfast cereal, Kellogg's	71	Now and then
Hummus, regular	6	A great alternative to butter

÷ average   ★ little or no carbs   ▼ high in saturated fat

FOOD	GI VALUE	
White sandwich bread	70	Take it easy
ICE CREAM		
Low-fat, vanilla	46	
Low-fat, chocolate	49	
Low-fat, with nuts	37	
Low-fat, rich vanilla	47	Indulgence food—energy dense,
Low-fat, toffee	37	so limit your serving size
Regular, full fat, average of several types	47÷▼	
Full fat, french vanilla	38▼	
Full fat, chocolate	37▼	
Instant mashed potato	69÷	Take it easy
Instant rice, white, cooked 6 min	87	Go slow
Ironman PR bar, chocolate	39	Snack bar
Jam, apricot fruit spread, reduced sugar	55	Enjoy in moderation
Jam, strawberry, regular	56÷	Enjoy in moderation
Jasmine rice, white, long-grain, cooked in rice cooker	109	Keep as an occasional treat
Jelly, diet	★	A low calorie alternative to regular jelly
Jelly beans	78÷	Go slow
Jevity, fiber-enriched drink	48	A nutrition supplement
Kaiser bread rolls, white	73	Go slow
Kavli Norwegian crispbread	71	Eat in moderation
Kidney beans, red, canned, drained	36÷	A convenient everyday food
Kidney beans, red, dried, boiled	28÷	A super food
Kidz, Heinz, Fruit Fingers, banana	61	Okay occasionally
Kiwi fruit, fresh	58	A good choice
Lamb	★	Keep it lean
Lean Cuisine, French–style Chicken with Rice	36	A low GI convenience meal
Lebanese bread, white	75	Take it easy
Leeks	★	An everyday food
Lentil soup, canned	44	A good choice
LENTILS		
Green, canned	48÷	
Green, dried, boiled	30÷	One of nature's superfoods
Lentils, red, dried, boiled	26÷	
Lettuce	★	An everyday food
Licorice, soft	78	Go slow
Life Savers, peppermint	70	An occasional treat
Light rye bread	68	A fair choice
Light soy milk, reduced-fat	44	A good choice
Lima beans, baby, frozen, reheated in microwave	32	An everyday food
Linguine pasta, thick, durum wheat, boiled	46÷	Serve with low-fat sauces
Linguine pasta, thin, durum wheat, boiled	52÷	Don't overcook—the GI will rise
Linseed and soy bread	55	Good for everyday eating

÷ average   ★ little or no carbs   ▼ high in saturated fat

FOOD	GI VALUE	
Liverwurst	▼★	High in saturated fat—use in small amounts
Low-fat frozen fruit dessert, mango	42	A good choice in moderation
Lungkow bean thread noodles, dried, boiled	33÷	A low-GI noodle
M&M's, peanut	33▼	Go slow
Macaroni, white, plain, boiled	47÷	Serve with low-fat sauces
Macaroni and cheese, made from packet mix, Kraft	64▼	Now and then
Malted Milk Powder, Nestlé, in whole milk	45▼	Once in a while
Mango, fresh	51÷	Enjoy on a regular basis when in season
Maple flavored syrup	68	Take it easy
Maple syrup, pure, Canadian	54	Use in moderation
Marmalade, orange	55÷	Enjoy in moderation
Mars Bar, regular	62▼	Indulgence food—go slow
Marshmallows, plain, pink and white	62	Occasional treat
McDonald's Vege Burger	59	Now and then
Melba toast, plain	70	Occasional use
Milk, condensed, sweetened	61▼	Go slow
MILK		
Low-fat, calcium enriched (1% fat) milk	23	All low GI—use lower fat varieties for weight control
Reduced-fat (1.4% fat) milk	30	
Skim, fat-free	32	
Whole milk (3.5 % fat)	÷ 27	
Milk, low-fat, chocolate, with aspartame	24	A better choice
Milk, low-fat, chocolate, with sugar	34	Enjoy in moderation
MILK CHOCOLATE		
Cadbury's Milk Chocolate, plain	49▼	Indulgence food
Dove, milk chocolate	45▼	
Plain milk chocolate, regular	41÷▼	
Plain milk chocolate, reduced sugar	35÷▼	
Plain, with fructose instead of regular sugar	20▼	
Nestlé plain milk chocolate	42▼	
Milky Bar, plain white chocolate, Nestlé	44▼	An occasional indulgence
Millet, boiled	71	Now and then
Minestrone soup, Campbell's	39	A healthy convenience food
Mint Mania Nutrition Bar	23	Snack bar
Morning Coffee biscuits	79▼	Go slow
MUESLI		
Muesli, gluten-free, with 1.5% fat milk	39	GI and fat content varies—choose lower saturated fat varieties
Muesli, low-fat	54	
Muesli, natural	49÷	
Muesli, Swiss, Alpen	55	
Muesli bar, crunchy with dried fruit	61	An occasional treat
Muesli bar, chewy with choc chips or fruit	54÷▼	Now and then

÷ average   ★ little or no carbs   ▼ high in saturated fat

FOOD	GI VALUE	
MUFFINS		
Apple muffin, home-made	46÷▼	
Blueberry, commercially made	59▼	Enjoy occasionally—
Bran, commercially made	60▼	choose lower fat types
Carrot, commercially made	62▼	
Oatmeal, made from packet mix	69▼	
Multigrain sandwich bread	65	Take it easy
Multigrain 9 grain bread	43	A good choice
Mung beans	39	A five-star food
Mung bean noodles (Lungkow bean thread), dried, boiled	33÷	A good choice
Mushrooms	★	An everyday food
Navy beans, cooked, canned	38÷	A star performer
Navy beans, dried, boiled	33÷	A star performer
Nectar, grape	52	An alternative to honey— use in moderation
Nesquik powder, chocolate, in 1.5% fat milk	41	Okay now and then
Nesquik powder, strawberry, in 1.5% fat milk	35	Okay now and then
Nestlé Chocolate Mousse	37	Great for a snack or dessert
Nestlé Diet Chocolate Mousse	37	A good choice
Nestlé Diet Crème Caramel	33	A good choice
Nestlé Diet Lemon Cheesecake	31	A good choice
New potato, unpeeled and boiled 20 min	78	Take it easy
New potato, canned, microwaved 3 min	65	A lower GI potato
NOODLES		
Dried rice, boiled	61	
Fresh rice, boiled	40	
Mung bean (Lungkow bean thread), dried, boiled	33÷	Try lower GI, lower fat types for everyday eating
Noodles, 99% fat-free	67	
Soba noodles, instant, served in soup	46	
Udon, plain	62	
Nutella, chocolate-hazelnut spread	33	Enjoy in moderation
Nutri-Grain, breakfast cereal	66	Take it easy
Oat bran, unprocessed	55÷	A useful source of fiber— add to oatmeal or cereal
Oat bran and honey bread	49	An everyday food
Oatmeal, instant, made with water	82	Go slow—use traditional oats instead
Oatmeal, made from steel-cut oats with water	52	Look for these at a health food shop
Oats, raw, rolled	59	A fair choice
Okra	★	An everyday food
Onions	★	An everyday food
Orange, fresh	42÷	Great anytime
Orange cordial, reconstituted	66	Drink occasionally

÷ average　★ little or no carbs　▼ high in saturated fat

FOOD	GI VALUE	
Orange juice, unsweetened	50÷	Drink in moderation
Oysters, natural, plain	★	Go for it!
Pancakes, prepared from mix	67▼	Enjoy as a special treat
Pancakes, buckwheat, gluten-free, made from packet mix	102	Take it easy
Papaya, fresh	56	A good choice
Parsnips	97	Modest servings are no problem
Party pies, beef, cooked	45▼	Go slow
PASTA		
Capellini, white, boiled	45	
Cheese tortellini, cooked	50	
Corn pasta, gluten-free, boiled	78	
Fettuccine, egg, boiled	40÷	
Linguine, thick, durum wheat, boiled	46÷	
Linguine, thin, durum wheat, boiled	52÷	
Macaroni, white, durum wheat, boiled	47÷	
Macaroni and cheese, from packet mix, Kraft	64	
Protein-enriched, boiled	28	
Ravioli, meat-filled, boiled	39	Chose lower-GI types
Rice and corn pasta gluten-free	76	for regular eating
Rice pasta, brown, boiled	92	
Rice vermicelli, dried, boiled, Chinese	58	
Spaghetti, gluten-free, canned in tomato sauce	68	
Spaghetti, protein-enriched, boiled	27	
Spaghetti, white, durum wheat, boiled 10–15 min	44÷	
Spaghetti, whole-wheat, boiled	42	
Spirali, white, durum wheat, boiled, Vetta	43	
Split pea and soya pasta shells, gluten-free, boiled	29	
Star Pastina, white, boiled 5 min	38	
Vermicelli, white, durum wheat, boiled	35	
Peach, canned, in heavy syrup	58	Okay; try those in natural juice
Peach, canned, in light syrup	57÷	Okay; try those in natural juice
Peach, canned, in natural juice	45	Enjoy when fresh aren't available
Peach, fresh	42÷	Great anytime
Peanuts, roasted, salted	14÷	A great snack, in moderation
Peanut Power Nutrition Bar	27	Snack bar
Pear, fresh	38÷	Great anytime
Pear halves, canned, in natural juice	44÷	A good choice
Pear halves, canned, in reduced-sugar syrup	25	Good with cereal or low-fat yogurt
Peas, dried, boiled	22	A nutritious food—add to stews and soups
Peas, green, frozen, boiled	48÷	An everyday food
Pecan nuts, raw	10	A great snack or recipe ingredient
Peppers, all types	★	Great anytime

÷ average   ★ little or no carbs   ▼ high in saturated fat

FOOD	GI VALUE	
Pineapple, fresh	59÷	A good choice
Pineapple juice, unsweetened	46	Enjoy in moderation—one glass a day
Pinto beans, canned, in brine	45	A nutritious convenience food
Pinto beans, dried, boiled	39	A star performer
Pita bread, white	57	A fair choice—try whole-wheat
PIZZA		
Super Supreme, pan, Pizza Hut	36▼	Go slow—occasional indulgence
Super Supreme, thin and crispy, Pizza Hut	30▼	
Vegetarian Supreme, thin and crispy, Pizza Hut	49▼	
Plum, raw	39÷	An everyday food
Polenta, boiled	68	Enjoy occasionally
Popcorn, plain, cooked in microwave	72÷	Skip the butter and make it a high-fiber snack
Pop-Tarts, double chocolate	70	Indulgence food
Pork	▼★	Eat it lean
Porridge, multigrain, made with water	55	A good choice—serve with lower fat milk
Potato chips, plain, salted	54÷▼	Indulgence food
POTATOES		
Instant mashed potato	88	All potatoes tend to be high GI—sweet potato can be substituted
New, canned, microwaved 3 min	65	
New, unpeeled, boiled 20 min	78	
Russet, baked without fat	77	
Sweet potato, baked	46÷	
Pound cake, plain	54▼	Indulgence food
Power Bar, chocolate	56÷	A nutrition supplement for serious sportspeople
POWDERED DRINKS		
Malted milk powder in full fat milk	37▼	Enjoy in moderation and use low-fat milk
Malted milk powder in reduced-fat milk	40▼	
Malted milk powder in skim milk	46▼	
Chocolate powder in full fat milk	33▼	
Chocolate powder in reduced-fat milk	36÷▼	
Chocolate powder in skim milk	39▼	
Pretzels, oven-baked, traditional wheat flavor	83	Take it easy; energy dense
Protein-enriched pasta, boiled	28	An excellent choice with low-fat sauce
Prunes, pitted, Sunsweet	29	A handful makes a great snack
Pudding, chocolate, instant, made from packet with whole milk	47÷▼	Okay occasionally—use low-fat milk
Pudding, vanilla, instant, made from packet mix and whole milk	40▼	Okay occasionally—use low-fat milk
Pudding, Sustagen, instant vanilla, made from powdered mix	27	A nutrition supplement
Puffed buckwheat cereal	65	Puffing grains increases their GI
Puffed crispbread, white	81	Go slow

÷ average   ★ little or no carbs   ▼ high in saturated fat

FOOD	GI VALUE	
Puffed rice cakes, white	82	An occasional snack
Puffed Wheat, breakfast cereal	80	Take it easy
Pumpernickel bread	50÷	An excellent choice
Pumpkin	75	Eat freely; low in carbs
Pure Canadian maple syrup	54	Use in moderation
Quinoa, organic, boiled	53	An excellent grain food
Radishes	★	An everyday food
Raisins	64	Enjoy in moderation
Ravioli, durum wheat flour, meat-filled, boiled	39▼	A good choice with a tomato-based sauce
RICE		
Arborio risotto rice, white, boiled	69	
Basmati rice, white, boiled	58	
Broken rice, Thai, white, cooked in rice cooker	86	
Glutinous rice, white, cooked in rice cooker	98	
Instant rice, white, cooked 6 min with water	87	Choose lower GI varieties for everyday eating
Jasmine rice, white, long-grain, cooked in rice cooker	109	
Quick cooking rice	80	
Rice, Uncle Ben's converted long grain, parboiled	38÷	A clever choice
Rice, Uncle Ben's long grain and wild	54	
Rice, brown	50	
Wild rice, boiled	57	
Rice Bran, extruded	19	A good source of fiber to add to cereal
Rice cakes, puffed, white	82	Go slow
Rice drink, natural, low-fat	92	Go slow
Rice Krispies, breakfast cereal, Kellogg's	82	Now and then
Rice milk	92	Go slow
Rice noodles, dried, boiled	61	Take it easy
Rice noodles, freshly made, boiled	40	A smart choice
Rice pasta, brown, gluten-free, boiled	92	Go slow
Rice vermicelli, dried, boiled	58	A fair choice
Rich Tea biscuits	55▼	Limit your intake
Risotto rice, Arborio, boiled	69	Enjoy in moderation
Roll (bread), Kaiser, white	73	Go slow
Roll-Ups, processed fruit snack	99	An occasional treat—fresh fruit is best
Russet potato, baked without fat	85÷	Take it easy
Rye	34	An excellent choice
Rye bread	51	An everyday food
Ryvita crispbread	69	Take it easy
Salami	▼★	Go slow—high in fat
Salmon	★	A fantastic food
Sardines	★	A good choice, fresh or canned in brine or water

÷ average   ★ little or no carbs   ▼ high in saturated fat

FOOD	GI VALUE	
Sausages, fried	28▼	Go slow—choose lean varieties
Scallops, natural, plain	★	Eat in moderation, avoid saturated fat in cooking
Scones, plain, made from packet mix	92	Special occasion food
Semolina, cooked	55÷	Good alternative to instant oatmeal
Sesame seeds	★	Nutritious but high in fat—use in moderation
Shallots	★	An everyday food
Shellfish (shrimp, crab, lobster, etc.)	★	Fantastic food
Shortbread biscuits	64▼	Indulgence food—high in saturated fat
Shredded Wheat breakfast cereal	75÷	Go slow
Skittles	70▼	A special treat
Slim-Fast Drink, can, vanilla or chocolate	39÷	A meal replacement drink
Slim-Fast Drink powder, all flavors, made with skim milk	35÷	A meal replacement drink
Snickers Bar, regular	41▼	Indulgence food
Snowpea sprouts	★	An everyday food
SOY PRODUCTS		
Light soy milk, reduced-fat (1.5%), calcium-fortified	44	Use in moderation
Original soy milk, full fat (3%)	44	
Soy milk, full fat (3%), calcium-enriched	36	A good choice
Soy yogurt, peach and mango, 2% fat	50	
Smoothie drink, banana, low-fat	30	
Smoothie drink, chocolate-hazelnut, low-fat	34	
Soba noodles, instant, served in soup	46	A good choice
SOFT DRINKS		
Coca-Cola	63	Save for special occasions
Diet varieties	★	
Fanta, orange soft drink	68	
SOUP		
Black bean, canned	64	Choose lower GI, low-fat varieties
Clear consommé, chicken or vegetable	★	
Green pea, canned	66	
Lentil, canned	44	
Split pea, canned	60	
Tomato, canned	45÷	
Traditional Minestrone, Campbell's	39	
Sourdough rye bread	48	An everyday food
Sourdough wheat bread	54	A good choice
SOY MILK		
Calcium-enriched, full fat	36	Choose lower fat types to limit your fat intake
Light, calcium-fortified, reduced-fat	44	
Original, full fat (3%)	44	

÷ average   ★ little or no carbs   ▼ high in saturated fat

FOOD	GI VALUE	
Soy smoothie drink, banana	30	Enjoy in moderation
Soy smoothie drink, chocolate-hazelnut	34	Now and then
Soy yogurt, peach and mango	50	Eat in moderation
Soybeans, canned	14	An excellent choice
Soybeans, dried, boiled	18÷	A five-star food
Spaghetti, gluten-free, canned in tomato sauce	68	Lower GI than other gluten-free pastas
Spaghetti, white, durum wheat, boiled 10–15 min	44÷	Serve with non-creamy sauces
Spaghetti, whole-wheat, boiled	42	An everyday food
Special K, regular, breakfast cereal, Kellogg's	56÷	A fair choice
Spelt multigrain bread	54	An everyday food
Spinach	★	An everyday food
Spirali pasta, white, durum wheat, boiled	43	An everyday food
Split pea soup	60	A fair choice
Split peas, yellow, boiled 20 min	32	Excellent—nutritious and versatile
Sponge cake, plain	46	An occasional treat
Spring onions	★	An everyday food
Squash, yellow	★	An everyday food
Squid or calamari, not battered or crumbed	★	Enjoy prepared in low-fat ways
Steak, any cut	▼★	Buy lean steak; grill or barbecue
Stoned Wheat Thins, crackers	67	For special occasions
Strawberry jam, regular	54÷	Enjoy in moderation
Strawberries, fresh	40	Any time you like
Stuffing, bread	74	Go slow
Sugar	68÷	Sugar can be a source of excess calories—go slow
Sunsweet pitted prunes	29	Great for snacks or with breakfast cereal
Super Supreme pizza, pan, Pizza Hut	36▼	Low GI but high saturated fat content—go slow
Super Supreme pizza, thin and crispy, Pizza Hut	30▼	Indulgence food
Sushi, salmon	48	A good choice
Sustagen drink, dutch chocolate	31	A nutrition supplement
Sustagen pudding, instant vanilla, made from powdered mix	27	A nutrition supplement
Sustagen Sport, milk-based drink	43	A nutrition supplement
Sweet corn, whole kernel, canned, drained	46	An everyday food
Sweet corn, on the cob, boiled	48	An everyday food
Sweet potato, baked	46÷	A low GI substitute for regular potato
Sweetened condensed whole milk	61▼	Go slow
Sweetened dried cranberries	64	Eat in moderation
Syrup, golden	63	Enjoy in sensible amounts— occasionally
Syrup, maple, pure Canadian	54	Use in moderation
Syrup, maple flavored	68	Take it easy

÷ average   ★ little or no carbs   ▼ high in saturated fat

FOOD	GI VALUE	
Taco shells, cornmeal-based, baked	68	Serve with filling made from lean mince
Tahini, pure	★	High in fat—use in small amounts
Tapioca, boiled, with milk	81	Go slow
Taro	54	A low GI substitute for potato
Tea, black or green, no milk or sugar	★	Any time you like
Tofu (bean curd), plain, unsweetened	★	Use low-fat cooking methods
Tomato juice, no added sugar	38	Drink in moderation
Tomato soup, canned	45÷	A good choice—serve with low-GI bread
Tortellini, cheese, boiled	50▼	In moderation
Tortilla, wheat	30	An everyday food
Tortilla, wheat, with pinto beans and tomato sauce	28	A good choice
Trout, fresh or frozen	★	Fantastic food
Tuna, fresh or canned in water or brine	★	Fantastic food
Turkey	▼★	Serve it lean without the skin
Twix bar	44▼	Indulgence food
Udon noodles, plain	62	Now and then
Vanilla cake made from packet mix with vanilla frosting, Betty Crocker	42▼	Indulgence food
Vanilla custard, reduced-fat	37	Good with fruit as a dessert
Vanilla pudding, instant, made from packet mix and whole milk	40▼	Now and then
Vanilla wafer cookies	77▼	Special treat
Veal	★	A nutritious food—eat it lean
Vege Burger, McDonald's	59	Go slow
Vegetarian Supreme Pizza, thin and crispy, Pizza Hut	49▼	Indulgence food
Vermicelli, white, durum wheat, boiled	35	An everyday food
Vinegar	★	Everyday food—great as a salad dressing
Wafers, vanilla, plain	77▼	Now and then
Waffles, plain	76▼	An occasional treat
Water crackers, plain	78	Special occasion food
Watercress	★	An everyday food
Watermelon, raw	76÷	No problem in moderation; low in carbs
Wheat, cracked, bulgur, ready to eat	48÷	Excellent in salads such as tabbouli
WHITE BREAD		
Kaiser rolls	73	
Lebanese bread, white	75	
Pita bread, white	57	Take it easy
Regular, sliced white bread, enriched	71÷	
Sandwich bread	70	
Wonder White, white bread	80	

÷ average   ★ little or no carbs   ▼ high in saturated fat

FOOD	GI VALUE	
WHOLE-WHEAT BREAD		
Whole-wheat, enriched wheat flour	70	Take it easy
Whole-wheat kernels	41	An excellent choice
Wild rice, boiled	57	
Wonder White, white bread	80	Go slow
Yam, peeled, boiled	37 ÷	A five-star food
YOGURT		
LOW-FAT YOGURT		
Apricot, mango and peach	26	Good for a snack
Berry	28	or dessert
French vanilla	26	
With fruit and artificial sweetener	14	A clever choice
FAT-FREE YOGURT		
Berry	38	Makes a good
French vanilla	40	snack or dessert
Mango	39	
Zucchini	★	An every day food

Choose lower fat types for everyday eating

DAILY FOOD, TELEVISION, AND ACTIVITY JOURNAL

Make three photocopies of this page and complete a three-day journal at frequent intervals (once a month to start with, then every three months in the first twelve months) to help you focus on your strengths and weaknesses.

Date _____

Meal	Time	Foods and drinks consumed *(indicate item and amount)*	Did you include			Situation How did you feel? (e.g. happy, sad, angry)
			Low-GI carbs?	Protein?	Good fats?	

TV duration (circle): 0   30   60   90   120   150   180   or more ___ minutes

Exercise type (check):   ☐ Aerobic   ☐ Resistance

Exercise duration (circle): 0   5   10   15   20   30   45   60   or more ___ minutes

Rate of perceived exertion (circle): 1   2   3   4   5   6   7   8   9   10

Further Resources

*T*he **following Web** sites offer responsible advice on food, health, and body weight; however, our listing of them does not signify endorsement.

CALORIE CONTROL COUNCIL
This Web site offers several weight-loss resources, including an exercise calculator, calorie counter, and recipes.
www.caloriecontrol.org

THE DIET CHANNEL
This Web site reviews popular diets and offers an abundance of diet tools, tips, and techniques.
www.thedietchannel.com

COLUMBIA SURGERY
This Web site offers information about surgery to aid weight loss.
www.columbiasurgery.org/divisions/obesity

NATIONAL WEIGHT CONTROL REGISTRY
University of Colorado Web site for the National Weight Control Registry.
www.nwcr.ws

AUSTRALASIAN SOCIETY FOR THE STUDY OF OBESITY
This Australian Web site is primarily for health professionals, but it offers reliable, scientific information about the causes, treatment, and prevalence of obesity with links to national policy.
www.asso.org.au

DIETCLUB

An Australian Web site with a wealth of information about food, nutrition, and weight management. It includes a database for looking up basic nutrient information on almost any food.
www.dietclub.com.au

DIETITIANS' ASSOCIATION OF AUSTRALIA

The Australian Dietitians' Association Web site, where you can look for a dietitian and learn some smart eating tips.
www.daa.asn.au

FOODWATCH

The Web site of Australian dietitian Catherine Saxelby, where you can have your questions about food answered and gain access to information, newsletters, recipes, and quizzes about food and nutrition.
www.foodwatch.com.au

GLYCEMIC INDEX RESEARCH SERVICE

The University of Sydney GI Web site, where you can learn about the GI and access the GI database.
www.glycemicindex.com

IF NOT DIETING THEN WHAT

Dr. Rick Kausman's Web site offers a different, but realistic, perspective on weight and eating behavior management.
www.ifnotdieting.com

NUTRITION AUSTRALIA

An Australian community-based Web site, providing information on food and physical activity to help people achieve optimum health. Includes publications for sale and links to related sites.
www.nutritionaustralia.org

Low-GI foods and weight:
a summary of the scientific evidence

Country	Subjects	Study design	Findings	Reference details
Australia	Overweight young adults	89 subjects followed 1 of 4 diets for 12 weeks: (1) standard low-fat; (2) low-GI; (3) higher protein; (4) low-GI and protein	Compared with the standard low-fat diet, all 3 modified diets produced around 50% more fat loss. Risk factors for heart disease improved more on the low-GI diet	McMillan-Price et al., unpublished findings, 2004.
USA	Overweight young adults	39 subjects consumed a low-GI or low-fat diet to achieve a 10% weight loss in both groups	Resting metabolic rate declined less in the low-GI group (-6%) than the low-fat group (-11%). Risk factors for heart disease improved more on the low-GI diet	Pereira et al., in press
USA	Overweight adolescents	16 subjects followed a low-fat diet or a low-glycemic load diet for 12 months	Those who followed the low-GL diet lost more body fat and kept it off. The low-fat group gained body fat during the second 6 months	Ebbeling et al., Archives of Pediatric and Adolescent Medicine, 2003
UK	Overweight men	17 men consumed 1 of 4 diets for 24 days	Despite efforts to maintain identical energy intake, men on the low-GI diet lost weight compared with those on the high-GI, high-fat and high-sugar diets	Byrnes et al., British Journal of Nutrition, 2003.

Sources

The diagram on page 5 is redrawn from *Pocket Picture Guide to Obesity* (1997) by I. D. Caterson and J. Broom. London: Excerpta Medica.

The diagram on page 20 is redrawn from S. H. A. Holt, J. C. Brand-Miller, and P. Petocz (1997): An insulin index of foods: Insulin demand generated by 1000 kJ portions of common foods. *American Journal of Clinical Nutrition* 66: 1264–76.

The diagram on page 25 is redrawn from D. S. Ludwig, J. A. Majzoub, A. Al-Zahrani, G. E. Dallal, I. Blanco, and S. B. Roberts (1999): High glycemic index foods, overeating, and obesity. *Pediatrics* 103: 3.

The diagram on page 27 (top) is redrawn from C. B. Ebbeling, M. M. Leidig, K. B. Sinclair, J. P. Hangen, and D. S. Ebbeling (2003): *Archives of Pediatric and Adolescent Medicine* 157: 725–27.

The extract on page 55 is from *Diary of a Fat Man* (2003) by Paul Jeffreys. Auckland: Penguin.

The information on stages of change on page 82 is adapted from J. O. Prochaska, C. C. DiClemente, and J. C. Norcross (1992): In search of how people change. *American Psychologist* 47: 1102–04.

Acknowledgments

A **book like** this doesn't get written without a great deal of outside help. Everyone at Hodder Headline Australia deserves a medal for professionalism, but we want to single out our editor, Siobhan Gooley, who gave it everything she had, and Lisa Highton, ever active and committed on our behalf, making the vital strategic decisions that have made the *New Glucose Revolution* series the success it is. We would be nowhere without our literary agent, Philippa Sandall, who shepherded us from start to finish and literally pulled us across the finishing line. Matthew Lore, our American publisher, inspired us and made sure we didn't forget the stress eaters and night-time eaters. We couldn't have done without Dr. Susanna Holt and the dedicated GI testing team, Vanessa de Jong, Hamilton Budd, Ellie Faramus, Emma Ryan, and all our cheerful, well-fed volunteers. We picked the brain of Professor Ian Caterson to distill the most up-to-date knowledge on the causes and treatment of obesity. Likewise, Professor Garry Egger (Professor Trim!) gave us his expertise on the role of exercise in weight-loss management. We thank Associate Professor David Ludwig at Boston Children's Hospital for his wise counsel and research on the GI and obesity. We are grateful to all the subjects who took part in our recent weight-loss trials—their efforts have strengthened our story and provided objective evidence of the benefits of following a low-GI diet. We would also like to thank Isa Hopwood, who "road-tested" the Action Plan. Finally, a big thank-you to all of our readers, colleagues, acquaintances, and clients for their inspiring feedback on how the GI has worked wonders for them. And of course we wouldn't have made it through so many late nights and working weekends without the loving support of our husbands, John Miller, Jonathan Powell, and Michael Price: a big hug and thank-you.

Index

The NEW GLUCOSE REVOLUTION Series—
BRINGING GOOD HEALTH TO MILLIONS

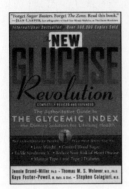

THE NEW GLUCOSE REVOLUTION

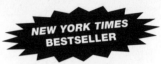

Written by the world's foremost authorities on the subject, whose findings are supported by hundreds of studies from Harvard University's School of Public Health and other leading research centers, *The New Glucose Revolution* shows how and why eating low-GI foods has major health benefits for everybody seeking to establish a way of eating for lifelong health. • **$15.95**

THE NEW GLUCOSE REVOLUTION COMPLETE GUIDE TO GLYCEMIC INDEX VALUES

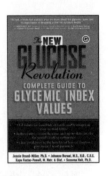

With GI values for hundreds of foods and beverages, *The New Glucose Revolution Complete Guide to Glycemic Index Values* makes it easier than ever to ascertain a food's GI value. Each of the three easy-to-read tables in this book lists a food's GI value, serving size, net carbohydrate per serving, and glycemic load, which is clearly explained. • **$6.95**

THE NEW GLUCOSE REVOLUTION LIFE PLAN

Both an introduction to the benefits of low-GI foods and an essential source for those already familiar with the concept, *The New Glucose Revolution Life Plan* presents the glycemic index within the context of today's full nutrition picture. With the glycemic index as its starting point, it gives readers clear guidelines for choosing the diet that is right for them. With the most authoritative, up-to-date and complete table of GI values published anywhere, *The New Glucose Revolution Life Plan* makes the glycemic index accessible and useful to more readers than ever before. • **$18.95**

THE NEW GLUCOSE REVOLUTION POCKET GUIDE TO THE TOP 100 LOW GI FOODS

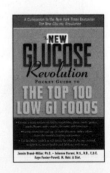

This handy A to Z guide offers in-depth entries for the top 100 foods with the lowest GI values. It covers each food's nutritional benefit and includes GI values, glycemic load, carbohydrate, fiber, and fat content, plus handy eating tips and a low-GI food finder. • **$6.95**

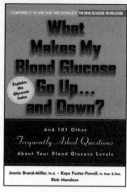

Answers the most frequently asked questions about your blood-glucose levels. • **$9.95**

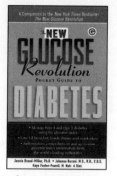

Help control your diabetes with low-GI foods. • **$6.95**

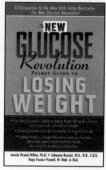

Eat yourself slim with low-GI foods. • **$6.95**

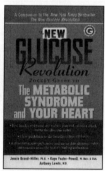

Healthy eating you can feel in your heart. • **$6.95**

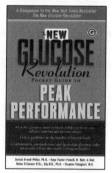

Eat to compete better than ever before. • **$6.95**

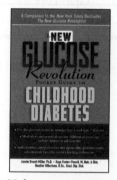

Help manage your child's diabetes with low-GI foods. • **$6.95**

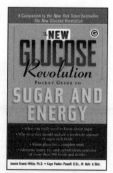

Sugar's off the black list—find out why. • **$6.95**

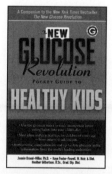

Raise healthy kids on low-GI foods. • **$6.95**

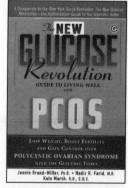

Use the glycemic index to beat your PCOS symptoms. • **$6.95**

Food manufacturers are showing increasing interest in having the GI values of their products measured. Some are already including the GI value of foods on food labels. As more and more research highlights the benefits of low-GI foods, consumers and dietitians are writing and telephoning food companies and diabetes organizations asking for GI data. This symbol has been registered in several countries, including the United States and Australia, to indicate that a food has been properly GI tested—in real people, not in a test tube—and also makes a positive contribution to nutrition. You can find out more about the program at www.gisymbol.com.au.

As consumers, you have a right to information about the nutrients and physiological effects of foods. You have a right to know the GI value of a food and to know it has been tested using appropriate standardized methodology.